Scalp Acupuncture and Clinical Cases

Jiao Shunfa

FOREIGN LANGUAGES PRESS   BEIJING

First Edition   1997

ISBN 7-119-01806-X

© Foreign Languages Press, Beijing, 1997

Published by Foreign Languages Press
24 Baiwanzhuang Road, Beijing 100037, China

Distributed by China International Book Trading Corporation
35 Chegongzhuang Xilu, Beijing 100044, China
P.O. Box 399, Beijing, China

Printed in the People's Republic of China

Scalp acupuncture, invented by Comrade Jiao Shunfa, started being popularized in March 1971. Thanks to its unique curative effect, it has quickly spread throughout the world and has become one of the common methods for China's urban and rural acupuncture doctors to treat cerebral diseases.

The invention of scalp acupuncture, which has opened up a new way for treating cerebral diseases, is of important significance to the study of tenets of acupuncture treatment.

I sincerely hope that the scalp acupuncture will be constantly perfected in practice and bring more benefits to the people.

HU XIMING
Chairman of the World Acupuncture and
Moxibustion Federation,
Vice-Minister of Public Health

November 14, 1990

Contents

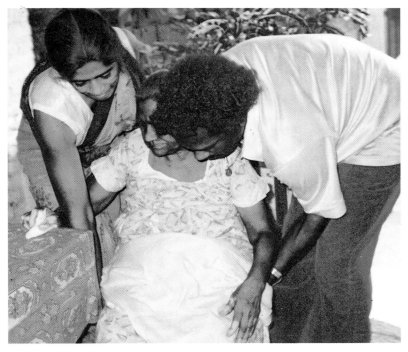

A patient from Pakistan with left hemiplegia due to cerebral thrombosis.

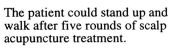

The patient could stand up and walk after five rounds of scalp acupuncture treatment.

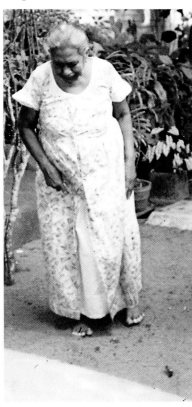

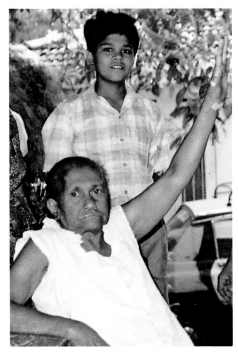

The left hand could be raised to the usual level.

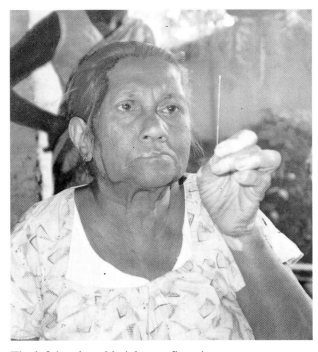

The left hand could pick up a fine pin.

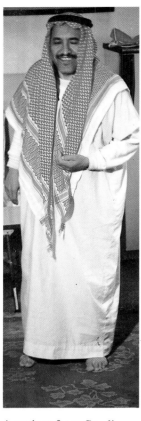

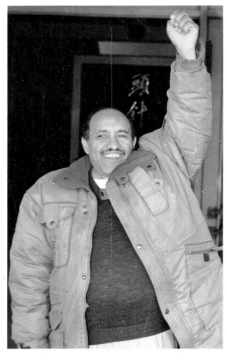

The left arm could extend and flex normally after 22 rounds of scalp acupuncture treatment.

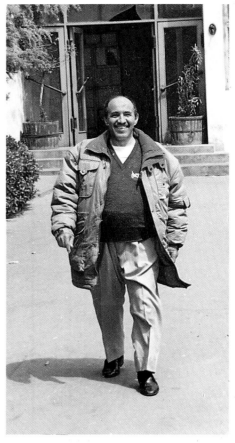

A patient from Saudi Arabia with left hemiplegic gait and half- flexed arm due to hemiplegia after cerebral thrombosis.

The hemiplegic gait of left leg was completely cured.

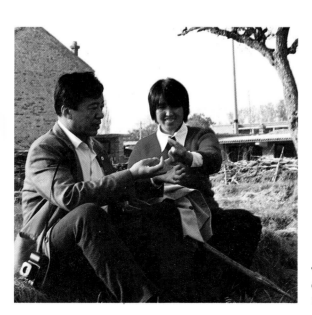

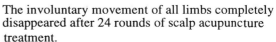

A patient from Jishan County with involuntary movement of limbs and unsteadiness lying on bed due to the chorea minor before treatment.

The involuntary movement of all limbs completely disappeared after 24 rounds of scalp acupuncture treatment.

FOREWORD

The scalp acupuncture is a therapy applied by needling the specific areas of the scalp to treat diseases. It is invented and developed by combining the theories and techniques of traditional acupuncture and the knowledge of modern physiology and anatomy of the nervous system on the basis of repeated scientific research and clinical practice for many years.

1. Inspiration from Theories and Techniques of Acupuncture

(1) Theories of Acupuncture

The theories of acupuncture may be traced back to the Spring and Autumn Period and Warring States Period (770-221 B.C.) and an integral theoretical system had been developed at that time, as evidenced in the *Internal Canon of the Yellow Emperor*.

In this ancient medical classic, fairly detailed descriptions can be found of the discovery of the meridian system, which is of vital importance to human life, and the peculiar invention of acupuncture that can cure many generalized diseases by localized stimulation.

The meridian system is the most important system in the human body; it can determine the survival or death of the patients, cure various diseases and adjust deficiency or excessiveness of human body. It is a huge network distributed all over the body to connect the internal organs with the external trunk and limbs and converges into the spinal cord and stops at the brain.

On the basis of thoroughly sorting out and carefully analysing the descriptions of meridians in ancient medical literature, one can divide the meridian system into the central and peripheral parts.

The central part comprises the brain and the spinal cord in the skull and spinal canal.

The spinal cord in spinal canal is also called Dumai (governor vessel), or the "sea" of all meridians and collaterals, or Shu (pivot); and the brain is considered the "sea" of Shu, or the centre of the meridian system.

According to the above statement, the governor vessel and the brain are the central part of the meridian system.

The peripheral part can be further divided into the part to connect the trunk and limbs and the part to connect the internal organs.

The part connecting the trunk and limbs comprises the meridians and collaterals from the brain and spinal cord and are distributed all over the trunk and limbs of the body, and the part linking the internal organs mainly refers to the Chongmai (thoroughfare vessel) and Renmai (conceptional vessel), which extend to the internal organs to control them. The thoroughfare vessel and the conceptional vessel go upward along the inner surface of spinal column as the "sea" of the meridian system, then emerge from the body and continue to go upward to converge at the throat. The thoroughfare vessel is the "sea" of the 12 meridians and the Renmai (conceptional vessel) is the "sea" of internal organs.

Besides the outlined descriptions of the meridians above, the ancient medical classics also contain descriptions and discussions of the meridian qi. As mentioned in *Miraculous Pivot*, "About the path of qi: The qi of chest, head, abdomen and legs all has its own path. The qi of the head flows to the brain; the qi of the chest flows to the shu acupoints in the breast and back; the qi of the abdomen flows to the shu acupoints in the back and meets with the thoroughfare vessel at the pulsating vessels beside the umbilicus; and the qi of the legs flows to Qijie (femoral artery at groins) and Chengshan (BL 57) above or below ankle," and "The Sijie (four paths) refers to the paths of circulating qi." From the discussions one can conclude: The ancient physicians already knew that the meridional qi of the head, chest, abdomen and legs each had its own path to flow, and that the qi of the head flew to brain. It indicates that the head and brain have a particular relationship with each other. Therefore, the acupuncture over the scalp should certainly produce a satisfactory therapeutic result. This forms the theoretical basis of scalp acupuncture used to treat diseases of the brain.

(2) Experience of Acupuncture Therapy

Besides important discussions on the meridian system, ancient medical literature also described in great detail acupuncture applied at the trunk and limbs to treat many general diseases. To apply needles over the scalp to treat diseases of the brain serves as an important example of acupuncture applied at meridians to treat the general diseases of the human body.

Another inspiration for the invention of scalp acupuncture is from the good therapeutic results obtained from stimulating the mu acupoints, which are the locations where the qi of internal organs converges and assembles. They are also taken as "special acupoints" used to treat diseases of the internal organs.

Each of the 12 internal organs has its specific mu point at the chest and abdomen region. They are the important acupoints to cure the diseases of their corresponding organs, although not all of them lie on the meridians related to their corresponding internal organs. The reason is that the mu points are all located over or close to their corresponding organs.

The mu point of stomach, Zhongwan (CV 12), 4 cun (unit of length used in acupuncture to locate the acupoints, equalling about 3 cm.) above the umbilicus, is an acupoint on Renmai conceptional vessel. Although it has no relation with the stomach meridian, it lies directly over the stomach.

The mu point of large intestine, Tianshu (ST 25), 2 cun laterally beside the umbilicus, is an acupoint on the stomach meridian. Although it has no relation with the large intestine meridian, it lies at a location on the body surface corresponding to the large intestine.

The mu point of pericardium, Danzhong (CV 17), right between the two nipples, is an acupoint on Renmai (conceptional vessel). Although it has no relation with the pericardium meridium, it lies at a location on the body surface corresponding to the pericardium.

The mu point of spleen, Zhangmen (LR 13), right below the tip of the 11th rib, is an acupoint on the liver meridian. Although it has no relation with the spleen meridian, it lies at a location on the body surface corresponding to the spleen.

The mu point of kidney, Jingmen (GB 25), right below the tip of the 12th rib, is an acupoint on the gallbladder meridian. Although it has no relation with the kidney meridian, it lies at a location on the body surface corresponding to the kidney.

The mu point of small intestine, Guanyuan (CV 4), 3 cun below the umbilicus, is an acupoint on the Renmai (conceptional vessel). Although it has no relation with the small intestine meridian, it lies at a location on the body surface corresponding to the small intestine.

The mu point of urinary bladder, Zhongji (CV 3), 4 cun below the umbilicus, is an acupoint on the Renmai (conceptional vessel). Although it has no relation with the urinary bladder meridian, it lies at a location on the body surface corresponding to the urinary bladder.

The mu point of Sanjiao (triple energizer), Shimen (CV 5), 2 cun below the umbilicus, is an acupoint of Renmai (conceptional vessel). Although it lies in the Xiajiao (lower energizer), not entirely correlated with all the three energizers, it may be used to treat diseases of the underlying reproductive and urinary organs.

In addition, the mu point of lung Zhongfu (LU 1), the mu point of liver Qimen (LR 14) and the mu point of gallbladder Riyue (GB 24) are all acupoints on their own meridians and lie on locations on the body surface corresponding to these organs themselves. Therefore, those mu points may produce more remarkable effects in treating diseases of the correlated organs than other acupoints on the corresponding meridians.

Now that better therapeutic results can be achieved by needling the mu points at the body surface corresponding to the internal organs to cure the diseases of these underlying organs, so better therapeutic results should also be made in treating cerebral diseases by needling stimulation applied at the corresponding locations of the scalp.

As proved by clinical practice, stimulating the acupoints at the head may produce satisfactory therapeutic effects in curing diseases of the brain; stimulating the acupoints in the chest and on the back may cure diseases of the chest, back and thoracic organs; stimulating the acupoints at the upper limbs may produce better cure of diseases of the upper limbs, head, face and thoracic organs; stimulating the acupoints at the abdominal, lumbar and sacral regions may cure diseases of those regions; and stimulating the acupoints of the lower limbs may cure diseases of the lower limbs and the abdominal, lumbar and sacral regions. This serves as an evidence to support the usage of scalp acupuncture to treat cerebral diseases and establishes an important principle for selecting acupoints in the acupuncture therapy.

2. Deciding Stimulation Areas over the Scalp According to the Functional Divisions of the Cerebral Cortex

The brain commands the various systems of the human body, including naturally the nervous system.

Ancient physicians in the Spring and Autumn Period and Warring States Period already got a profound understanding of the brain. For instance, *Miraculous Pivot* says, "The brain is the 'sea' (reservoir) of the spinal cord"; and "The blood and qi of the 12 meridians and 365 collaterals all go upward to the face and pass across the orifices of sensory organs." This indicates the ancients already knew that the brain was an organ where the blood and qi of all the organs and meridians converge and assemble.

Besides, the physicians at that time already began to study the functional divisions of the cerebral cortex. As mentioned in *Miraculous Pivot*, "The injury of left corner (of the head) may cause dysfunction of the right foot." It proves that the ancient physicians already knew the injury of left frontal and parietal region of the head may cause a dysfunction of the right foot. Of course, the injury referred to here is not limited to the superficial scalp, because the dysfunction of the right foot may not occur if the brain is not injured. It also serves as an evidence of the fact that the ancient physicians already knew the movement of the limb on one side is controlled by the brain on the opposite side and the limb may be paralysed when the brain is damaged.

In modern medicine, scientific study of the brain has produced many important achievements and the functional division of the cerebral cortex is one of them. The different areas of the cerebral cortex may play different functions. For example, the precentral gyrus may receive and analyze the sensation of contralateral limbs; and the speech, auditory and visual sensation all have their own controlling areas on the cerebral cortex.

The ancient physicians found that stimulating the scalp with needles produced therapeutic effects for diseases of the brain, and modern medicine has proved that the different areas of the cerebral cortex play different special functions. Therefore, the author got the idea to locate different stimulating areas over the scalp according to the functional divisions of the cerebral cortex and to stimulate those areas with needles for treatment of lesions at the corresponding parts of the brain.

3. Experimental Study and Clinical Evidence

(1) Experimental Study

The acupuncture therapy was discovered and developed from past clinical practice and will be proved by practice now and in the future, as said in *Miraculous Pivot*, "The therapeutic methods were developed in the past and are proved at present."

According to the experience of ancient physicians, Deqi (getting qi) is an important prerequisite of acupuncture therapy for obtaining a good therapeutic result. If the needling sensation reaches the lesion, a better therapeutic effect can be produced.

The author believed that if the needling sensation reached a paralysed limb, the needling stimulation at the scalp should then produce some therapeutic effect in curing the paralysis of the limb.

At the beginning, the author tried on himself for many times and found that the needling stimulation on the head could only produce a local sensation, but no sensation reached the limbs. Although he was slightly disappointed, he did not give up and stop the experiment. He thought that the conditions of various individuals are different and they may produce different responses to the needling stimulation. Failure to make the needling sensation reach the desired spot on himself does not necessarily mean it would also fail on other persons. Therefore, the author tried to carry on the study on his patients.

Once, he treated a patient with headache by applying needling stimulation at his right frontal region of the head , the patient said: "I have got a hot sensation on my left cheek." It was just like a sparkle that kindled the author's hope again and drove away his disappointment.

According to former clinical experience, the needling stimulation on one side of the body is commonly used to treat the lesions on the same side. This time, the patient detected a hot sensation on the opposite cheek. This showed the special relationship between the contralateral spread of the needling sensation and the crossed innervation of the brain cortex. The event gave the author encouragement to continue his study.

Once again, the author applied needling stimulation on the scalp of another patient. Likewise, it evoked a hot sensation in the limb on the other side. Ever since, the same phenomenon had been repeatedly observed in other patients. All these have provided a basis for the author to find more clinical evidence.

(2) Clinical Evidence

One day in August of 1970 when the author had dinner in a farmer's family in Jishan County, he heard the moan from an old woman, the 70-year-old mother of the host. She had suffered spasmodic pain in the arms and legs for years and tried different therapies to no avail. Physical examination made me believe that cerebral arteriosclerosis was the cause of her spasmodic pain and scalp acupuncture was applied over the postcentral gyrus. On the second day, the old woman stopped groaning and told the author that she felt much better.

In December 1970, the author was invited to visit a family in Jishan County for treating a woman with hemiplegia and she was confined to bed for more than 40 days. Physical examination showed that the patient was fully conscious, her tongue was slightly deviated to the right side, her right arm was completely paralysed, and her right leg was partially paralysed and could only raise up for 10 centimetres. With the aid of laboratory examinations, the author concluded that the hemiplegia of her right limbs was caused by cerebral syphilitic endarteritis.

Based on the diagnosis, the author inserted three needles into the scalp over the left precentral gyrus of the cerebral cortex. After quickly manipulating the needles, the patient felt a hot sensation in her paralysed limbs spreading from the proximal ends to the hand and foot tips. Having manipulated needles three times, the needles were removed. The patient was then asked to try to raise her arm. She did it and raised the right arm over the head fairly easily and the right leg could be extended and raised higher. Both the doctor and patient were overjoyed. The patient was encouraged to stand up to test her muscular strength. She did as asked. She could not only stand erect but also walk over a few steps without any support from others.

Although the doctor knew that needling stimulation at the scalp over the precentral gyrus may be effective to patients with hemiplegia, it was beyond his expectation that it could produce such unexpected excellent result. After just one treatment, the patient could stand up and walk despite the fact that the patient had been confined to bed for over 40 days.

On the second day of the first lunar month, 1971, the author was invited to visit the home of a friend in Jishan County for treating a 64-year-old woman who had contracted aphasia and paralysis in the right limbs. Diagnosis confirmed that she got cerebral thrombosis and three needles were inserted into the scalp over the left precentral gyrus. The needles were manipulated three times to produce stimulation. Before the needles were removed, the patient could already able to speak clearly, raise the affected arm to touch her head with her hand, and extend and bend the right leg. The treatment was given once a day for four more days. Then she could get up from bed to walk and take care of herself.

Repeated experience proves that needling stimulation at the scalp over the postcentral and precentral gyruses is effective to treat sensory and motor disturbance caused by cerebral arteriosclerosis or cerebral thrombosis, because the postcentral gyrus is the sensory area of the cerebral cortex to control the sensation of human body, and the precentral gyrus is the motor area to control the movement.

The news that good therapeutic results had been achieved with needling stimulation at scalp to cure paralysis was soon spread in and around Jishan County. More and more patients came to the author for help. He has not confined himself to treating paralysis only, but offered treatment to many other diseases. With the accumulation of clinical experience, the author tried to, besides the precentral and postcentral areas, define several new stimulating areas closely in line with the different functional areas of the cerebral cortex for treating various neurological disorders. Extensive and repeated clinical applications have proved that needling stimulation at the scalp over the different functional areas of the cerebral cortex is also effective in treating the symptoms and physical signs of cerebral lesions other than paralysis in most patients.

Later, according to the principle of the spread of the needling sensation and the therapeutic effects, the author defined the different stimulating areas for the internal organs over the frontal region of the scalp, including the thoracic cavity area, stomach area, and liver and gallbladder area.

In February 1972, the author made a systematical summary of the clinical data and named this new therapeutic technique "scalp acupuncture."

Scalp acupuncture quickly aroused the attention of the medical circles and won much acclaim from the patients. On March 18, 1971, a nominating meeting was held by the Yuncheng Prefectural Public Health Administration in Jishan County. Officials from the Public Health Administration of Shanxi Province attended the meeting. The author handed his paper to the Shanxi Provincial Public Health Administration and the Ministry of Public Health together with a recommendation letter from the Jishan County People's Hospital.

The officials of the provincial and prefectural public health administrations visited the Jishan County People's Hospital to meet patients treated with scalp acupuncture right after they had read the materials.

Having received the author's paper and the recommendation letter, the Ministry of Public Health sent an investigation group, formed by experts from the China Academy of Traditional Chinese Medicine to the Jishan County People's Hospital to make an evaluation of the scalp acupuncture. After the investigation, the group submitted a report to the Ministry of Public Health to ascertain the reliability of scalp acupuncture and affirm that Dr. Jiao Shunfa, the author of this book, as the inventor. In March and May of 1972, the Ministry of Public Health decided to run two training classes in scalp acupuncture in Jishan County to spread scalp acupuncture therapy throughout the country.

CHAPTER 1
STIMULATING AREAS

Ancient Chinese physicians discovered the nervous system in human body 2,500 years ago. At that time, it was called meridian system (meridians and collaterals). It is a huge and complicated system to connect the internal organs and the external trunk and limbs; and all the meridians converge into the spinal cord (spinal canal) and end at the brain. The meridian system can affect and determine the survival or death of human beings, be used to treat hundreds of diseases and adjust the deficiency and excessiveness of the human body. Judging by descriptions of the meridian system in the ancient medical literature, *Internal Canon of the Yellow Emperor*, compiled in the Spring and Autumn Period and Warring States Period, it is similar to the nervous system in modern medicine. I think the nervous system in modern medicine is derived from the meridian system through many transformations and modifications.

Therefore, the nervous system in human body was first discovered by Chinese people and the anatomy and physiology of nervous system in modern medicine is actually an inheritance and development of the ancient meridian system.

The scalp acupuncture was invented and developed through clinical practice by combining the techniques of traditional acupuncture and the knowledge of modern anatomy and physiology. The stimulating areas over the scalp are defined chiefly according to the location of the functional areas of the cerebral cortex. For example, since the precentral gyrus is a motor centre of the cerebral cortex, this area over the scalp is defined as the motor area.

I. Location and Function of Stimulating Areas

To define the stimulating areas, it is necessary to establish marking lines over the scalp according to some demarcations on the surface of the skull (Fig. 1-1).

Anterio-posterior median line: This median line is drawn from the midpoint between the eyebrows to the lower border of external occipital tuberosity.

Supraciliary-occipital line: This line is drawn from the midpoint of upper border of eyebrow to the tip of external occipital tuberosity.

(1) Motor area

Location: The upper end of motor area lies 0.5 cm behind the midpoint of anterio-posterior median line and the lower end lies at the intersect of the supraciliary-occipital line and anterior border of temple (Fig. 1-2).

Function:

1) Upper one-fifth: To treat paralysis of the contralateral lower limb.

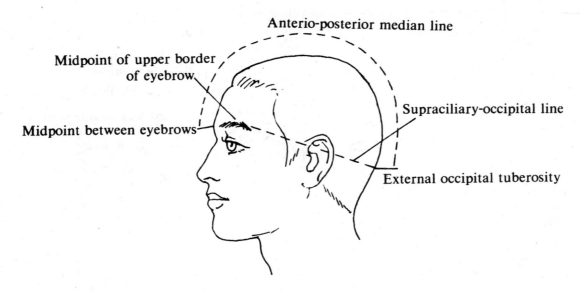

Fig. 1-1   Marking Lines of Skull

2) Middle two-fifths: To treat paralysis of the contralateral upper limb.

3) Lower two-fifths (first speech area): To treat facial paralysis, motor aphasia, dripping of saliva and disturbance of phonation.

(2) Sensory area

Location: It is parallel to and 1.5 cm behind the motor area (Fig. 1-3).

Function:

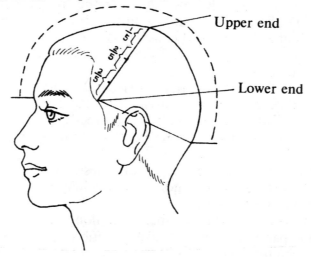

Fig. 1-2   Location of Motor Area

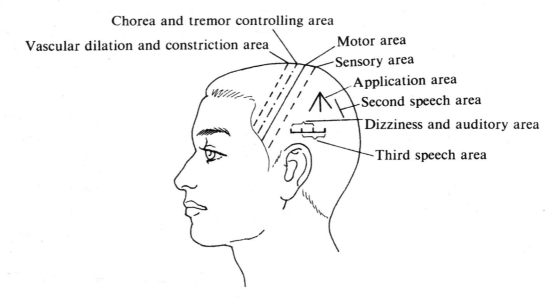

Fig. 1-3   Lateral View of Stimulating Areas on Scalp

1) Upper one-fifth: To treat pain, numbness and abnormal sensation of the contralateral side in the back and leg, occipital headache, pain of the neck and nape, and tinnitus.

2) Middle two-fifths: To treat pain, numbness and abnormal sensation of the contralateral arm.

3) Lower two-fifths: To treat numbness and pain of the contralateral side in the head and face.

(3) Controlling area of chorea and tremor

Location: It is parallel and 1.5 cm to the front of the motor area (Fig. 1-3).

Function: To treat involuntary movement and tremor of contralateral limbs.

(4) Vascular dilation and constriction area

Location: It is parallel and 1.5 cm to the front of the chorea and tremor controlling area (Fig. 1-3).

Function: To treat essential hypertension and cortical edema.

(5) Dizziness and auditory area

Location: Taking the point 1.5 cm directly above the tip of ear auricle as the midpoint of a horizonal line, which is 4 cm in length. This is the dizziness and auditory area (Fig. 1-3).

Function: To treat ipsilateral dizziness, tinnitus, auditory vertigo, cortical impairment of hearing and auditory hallucination.

(6) Second speech area

Location: To draw a parallel line along the anterio-posterior median line through the parietal tuber and take a section of 3 cm in length from the point 2 cm behind the tuber (Fig. 1-3).

Function: To treat anomic aphasia.

(7) Third speech area

Location: To draw an extending line backward from the midpoint of dizziness and auditory area, 4 cm in length (Fig. 1-3).

Function: To treat sensory aphasia.

(8) Application area

Location: To draw a line from parietal tuber to the centre of mastoid process and draw two more lines from the same origin of the first line at the tuber, one in front of the first line and another one behind the first line with an angle of 40 degree between the first line and each of the latter lines, all 3 cm in length (Fig. 1-3).

Function: To treat parectropia.

(9) Motor and sensory area of foot

Location: To draw two parallel lines 1 cm beside the anterio-posterior median line, 3 cm in length, from a point 1 cm to the front of the upper end of motor area to a point 1 cm to the back of the upper end of sensory area (Fig. 1-4).

Function: To treat pain, numbness and paralysis of the contralateral side of the back and contralateral leg. To treat bed-wetting of babies, cortical frequent micturition, cortical dysuria, cortical incontinence of urination and prolapse of anus by needling stimulation on both sides. To treat frequent and urgent urination due to acute cystitis, thirst, diuresis and increase of water intake due to diabetes mellitus, impotence, emission and prolapse of uterus by needling stimulation on both sides of the reproductive area and this area; to treat irritable colon and diarrhoea due to some other causes by needling stimulation on both sides of the intestine area and this area; to treat oliguria due to rheumatic heart disease by stimulating both sides of the thoracic cavity area and this area; and to treat hyperplasia syndrome of cervical and lumbar vertebrae, contact dermatitis and

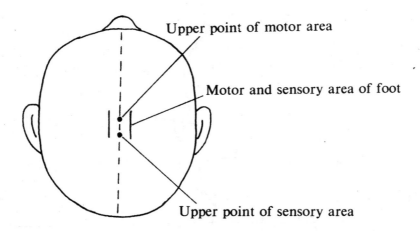

Upper point of motor area

Motor and sensory area of foot

Upper point of sensory area

Fig. 1-4   Stimulating Areas Viewed from the Top of the Head

neurodermatitis by stimulating both sides of the upper two-fifths of the sensory area and this area.

Frequent micturition, difficult urination and incontinence of urination caused by the functional disturbance of paracentral lobule due to cerebral arteriosclerosis with deficiency of blood supply in the anterior cerebral artery, cerebral thrombosis or other causes are named as "cortical frequent urination," "cortical difficult urination" and "cortical incontinence of urine" respectively.

(10) Optic area

Location: To draw two 4-cm parallel lines one centimetre beside the anterio-posterior median line, one on each side, from the level of external occipital tuberosity upward (Fig. 1-5).

Function: To treat cortical impairment of vision and cataract.

(11) Balance area

Location: To draw two parallel lines, 4 cm long vertically and 3.5 cm beside the median line on both sides, from the level of external occipital tuberosity downward (Fig. 1-5).

Function: To treat disturbance of body balance due to injury of the cerebellum.

(12) Stomach area

Location: To draw two parallel vertical lines of 2 cm in length directly above the centre of pupils from the anterior hair border (or 6 cm from the level of the midpoint between eyebrows) (Fig. 1-6).

Function: To treat the acute and chronic gastritis and pain due to peptic ulcer of stomach and duodenum.

(13) Liver and gallbladder area

Location: To extend the stomach area downward for 2 cm (Fig. 1-6).

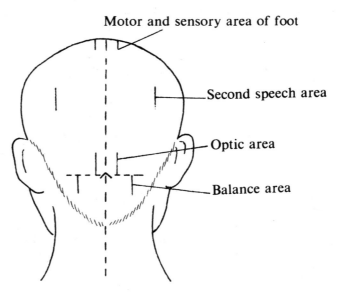

Fig. 1-5   Backside View of Stimulating Areas

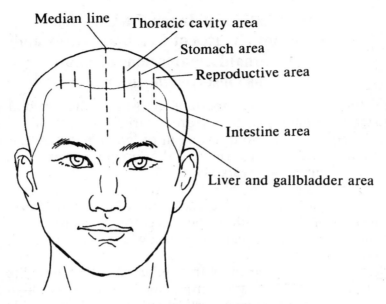

Fig. 1-6   Frontal View of Stimulating Areas

Function: To treat pain in the right upper abdomen due to disorders of the liver and gallbladder.

(14) Thoracic cavity area

Location: To draw two 4-cm parallel lines between median line and the stomach area on both sides, with 2 cm above and 2 cm below the anterior hairline (Fig. 1-6).

Function: To treat allergic asthma, bronchitis, angina pectoris, rheumatic heart disease, paroxysmal supraventricular tachycardia (also effective to some extent to treat palpitation, shortness of breath, edema and oliguria).

(15) Reproductive area

Location: To draw two 2-cm vertical lines, parallel from the frontal corner upward (Fig. 1-6).

Function: To treat functional uterine bleeding. To treat frequent urination and urgent urination due to acute cystitis, extreme thirst, polyuria and increase of water intake due to diabetes mellitus, and impotence, emission and prolapse of uterus by stimulating both sides of the motor and sensory area of foot and this area.

(16) Intestine area

Location: To extend the reproductive area on both sides downward for 2 cm (Fig. 1-6).

Function: To treat pain in the lower abdomen with certain effect.

The locations of frontal stimulating areas are defined according to the spread of the needling sensation and therapeutic effects, rather than according to the division of the underlying functional areas of the cerebral cortex.

II. Relations Between the Location of
Important Gyruses of Cerebral Cortex and
External Demarcations of Skull
as Observed in Autopsy

The relations between the important gyruses of the cerebral cortex and the anterio-posterior median line, motor area, parietal tuber and tip of auricle was studied in the anatomy of two cadavers in order to better define the stimulating areas according to the related gyruses of the cerebral cortex.

Autopsy (1): A girl of six years old

The anterior and posterior borders of the precentral gyrus lie at two points measured 13.2 cm and 15.3 cm respectively from the anterior end of anterio-posterior median line. The width of the precentral gyrus is 2 cm in the upper part and is 0.5 cm in the narrowest part, 4 cm below the median line. The length of the gyrus is 7 cm.

The Broca's area is basically a triangular area that lies directly below and slightly to the anterior side of the central sulcus; it is 2.8 cm high and 2 cm wide from front to back at the base. A vertical sulcus parallel with the central sulcus passes through the mid-line of the triangular area.

The width of the upper part of the central sulcus was 0.3 cm and the widest part of the sulcus was 0.8 cm; at the narrowest part the precentral and postcentral gyruses were overlapped with each other. The anterior and posterior borders of the upper end of the central sulcus lie at two points respectively, 15.3 cm and 15.6 cm behind the anterior end of the anterio-posterior median line.

The postcentral gyrus is 9 cm long; it is 1.5 cm wide at the upper end and 1.8 cm at the lower end. The anterior and posterior borders at the upper end rest at two points respectively, 15.6 cm and 16.9 cm behind the anterior end of the anterio-posterior median line.

The top of the supramarginal gyrus lies directly underneath the parietal tuber, being 3 cm long vertically and 2.5 cm wide laterally backward and the base is 1.2 cm in width.

The upper border of angular gyrus is 2 cm below the parietal tuber in parallel with the anterio-posterior median line, 3 cm long and 1.6 cm wide, and the base is 3 cm wide.

The upper and lower borders of superior temporal gyrus lie 1.6 cm and 0.7 cm above the tip of the ear respectively and the width of this gyrus is 0.7 to 1.0 cm (Table 1-1).

Autopsy (2): A man of 50 years old

The length of the anterio-posterior median line was 33 cm with the midpoint at 16.5 cm from the anterior end.

The anterior and posterior borders of the precentral gyrus lie at two points, 14 cm and 18.5 cm behind the anterior end of the anterio-posterior median line respectively. The length of this gyrus is 11 cm and the width of its lower end is 0.6 cm. The narrowest part is 0.5 cm wide and it is the part connecting the precentral and postcentral gyruses.

**Table 1-1. Relations Between Stimulating Areas and Important Gyruses
as Observed in Autopsy of the Six-Year-Old Girl**

Gyri of cerebral cortex	Location	Stimulating areas	Location	Correspondence
Anterioposterior median line	28.0 cm in length			
Midpoint of median line	14.0 cm from anterior end of median line			
Anterior border of precentral gyrus	13.2 cm from anterior end of median line	Motor area	14.5 cm from anterior end of median line	Good
Posterior border of precentral gyrus	15.3 cm from anterior end of median line			
Anterior border of postcentral gyrus	15.6 cm from anterior end of median line	Sensory area	16.0 cm from anterior end of median line	Good
Posterior border of postcentral gyrus	16.9 cm from anterior end of median line			
Supramarginal gyrus	Beneath parietal tuber	Application area	From parietal tuber downward	Good
Angular gyrus, 3 cm in length	2.0 cm below parietal tuber	Second speech area	2.0 cm below parietal tuber	Good
Upper border of superior temporal gyrus	1.6 cm above tip of ear	Dizziness and auditory area	1.5 cm below tip of ear	Good
Lower border of superior temporal gyrus	0.7 cm above tip of ear			

The Broca's area lies below and to the anterior side of the precentral gyrus; it is 3 cm high and its base is 2.5 cm wide.

The upper end of central sulcus situates 18.5 cm behind the anterior end of median line with a width of 0.2 cm. At most points of the central sulcus, the precentral and postcentral gyruses overlap each other.

The postcentral gyrus is 11 cm long and the widest segment is the lower part of the gyrus, 2.5 cm wide. The anterior and posterior borders of the upper end of this gyrus lie at the 18.5 cm and 20 cm points respectively behind the anterior end of median line, which means the upper end this gyrus is 1.5 cm wide.

The upper end of supramarginal gyrus lies underneath the parietal tuber, with one border going downward to the front side for 3.5 cm toward the tip of the ear and another border going downward and to the back side for 3.2 cm to make an 45-degree angle with the median line. The gyrus is 3.0 cm high and 1.2-1.5 cm wide.

The angular gyrus is in the deep part and 3 cm below the top side of the supramarginal gyrus; it is 1.7 cm high and 4 cm wide.

The superior temporal gyrus is 1.8 cm wide; its upper border and lower borders are 2.6 cm and 0.8 cm away from the tip of the ear respectively (Table 1-2).

**Table 1-2. Relations Between Stimulating Areas and Important Gyruses
as Observed in Autopsy of the 50-Year-Old Man**

Gyri of cerebral cortex	Location	Stimulating areas	Location	Correspondence
Anterioposterior median line	33.0 cm in length			
Midpoint of median line	16.5 cm from anterior end of median line			
Anterior border of precentral gyrus	14.0 cm from anterior end of median line	Motor area	17.0 cm from anterior end of median line	Good
Posterior border of precentral gyrus	18.5 cm from anterior end of median line			
Anterior border of postcentral gyrus	18.5 cm from anterior end of median line	Sensory area	18.5 cm from anterior end of median line	Good
Posterior border of postcentral gyrus	16.9 cm from anterior end of median line			
Supramarginal gyrus	Beneath parietal tuber	Application area	From parietal tuber downward	good
Angular gyrus, 3 cm in length	2.0 cm below parietal tuber	Second speech area	2.0 cm below parietal tuber	Good
Upper border of superior temporal gyrus	1.6 cm above tip of ear	Dizziness and auditory area	1.5 cm below tip of ear	good
Lower border of superior temporal gyrus	0.7 cm above tip of ear			

According to data obtained from the two cadavers, the important stimulating areas are all located over the functional areas of the corresponding gyruses.

Table 1-3. Location and Indications of Stimulating Areas of Scalp Acupuncture

NAME	LOCATION	INDICATION
Motor area	The upper end lies on the anterioposterior median line 0.5 cm behind	The upper one-fifths is used to treat paralysis of the contralateral leg; the middle

	its midpoint and the lower end lies at the intersect of supraciliary-occipital line and anterior border of temple. The connecting line of these two points is the motor area which can be divided into five sections.	two-fifths to treat paralysis of the contralateral arm; and lower two-fifths to treat paralysis of the contralateral side of the face, motor aphasia, dripping of saliva and impairment of phonation.
Sensory area	Parallel to and 1.5 cm behind the motor area.	Upper one-fifth: pain, numbness and abnormal sensation of the contralateral side of the back and the contralateral leg, occipital headache and tinnitus. Middle two-fifths: pain, numbness and abnormal sensation of the contralateral arm. Lower two-fifths: numbness and pain of the contralateral side of the head, migraine and arthritis of remporomandibular joint.
Chorea and tremor controlling area	Parallel to and 1.5 cm to the front of the motor area.	Involuntary movement and tremor of the contralateral limbs.
Vascular dilation and constriction area	Parallel to and 1.5 cm to the front of the chorea and tremor controlling area.	Essential hypertension and cortical edema.
Dizziness and auditory area	A horizontal line with its midpoint 1.5 cm directly above the tip of the ear auricle.	Ipsilateral dizziness, tinnitus, auditory vertigo, cortical impairment of hearing and auditory hallucination.
Second speech area	A 3-cm line parallel to the anterio-posterior median line, which goes downward from the point 2 cm behind the parietal tuber.	Anomic aphasia.
Third speech area	A horizontal line which goes 4 cm backward from the midpoint of the dizziness and auditory area.	Sensory aphasia.
Application area	Three lines, 3 cm in length each, drawn from the parietal tuber. The middle line goes toward the centre of mastoid process, the second line is to the front of the middle line and the third to the back, and together they make a 40-degree angle with the middle line.	Contralateral parectropia.
Motor and sensory area of foot	A parallel line of 3 cm in length over the vertex of the head and 1 cm beside the anterio-posterior median line, going from the 1-cm point to the anterior side of the upper end of the motor area to the 1-cm point to the posterior side of the upper end of the sensory area.	Pain, numbness and paralysis of the contralateral side of the back and contralateral leg. Baby bed-wetting, cortical frequent urination, cortical dysuria, cortical incontinence of urination and prolapse of anus by needling stimulation one both sides; frequent and urgent urination due to acute cystitis, thirst, polyuria and increase of water intake due to diabetes mellitus, impotence, emission and prolapse of uterus, and diarrhoea due to irritable colon or other diseases by simultaneous needling stimula-

		tion of the reproductive area and this area on both sides; oliguria due to rheumatic heart diseases by simultaneous needling stimulation of the thoracic cavity area and this area on both sides; hyperosteogeny of the cervical and lumbar vertebrae, alopecia areata, contact dermatitis, neurodermatitis and severe insomnia by simultaneous needling stimulation of the upper two-fifths of the sensory area and this area.
Optic area	A parallel line of 4 cm in length one centimetre beside the anterio-posterior median line, which goes upward from the level of the external occipital tuberosity.	Cortical impairment of vision and cataract.
Balance area	A vertical line of 4 cm in length and 3.5 cm beside the anterio-posterior median line, which goes downward from the level of external occipital tuberosity.	Disturbance of balance due to injury of the cerebellum.
Stomach area	A 2-cm vertical line which goes upward from the level of anterior hairline and runs parallel with the anterio-posterior median line and directly above the centre of the pupil.	Pain due to acute and chronic gastritis or peptic ulcer of the stomach and duodenum.
Liver and gall-bladder area	A 2-cm line extending downward from the stomach area and in parallel with the anterio-posterior median line.	Pain in the right upper abdomen due to disorders of the liver and gallbladder.
Thoracic cavity area	A 4-cm vertical line right between the anterio-posterior median line and the stomach area, with 2 cm above and 2 cm below the anterior hairline.	Allergic asthma, bronchitis, angina pectoris, chest distress, paroxysmal supraventricular tachycardia and shortness of breath.
Reproductive area	A 2-cm vertical line going upward from the frontal corner in parallel with the anterio-posterior median line.	Functional uterine bleeding; frequent and urgent urination due to acute cystitis, thirst, diuresis and increase of water intake due to diabetes mellitus, and impotence, emission and prolapse of uterus by simultaneous needling stimulation of the motor and sensory area of foot and this area on both sides.
Intestine area	A 2-cm vertical line extending further downward from the reproductive area.	Pain of the lower abdomen.

CHAPTER 2
TECHNIQUES OF ACUPUNCTURE AND OBSERVATION ON NEEDLING SENSATION

Acupuncture technique is an important factor affecting the therapeutic results. Good acupuncture technique should produce better therapeutic results, cause less side effects and sufferings to the patients, and is highly efficient.

According to above criteria and after repeated clinical practice, a desirable technique of scalp acupuncture, the "three-quickness acupuncture technique," was developed by the author. It will be described in great detail follow.

Section 1 Techniques of Acupuncture

I. Structure and Types of Acupuncture Needles

Commonly used acupuncture needles nowadays are made of stainless steel, and the handles are wrapped by winding thin copper wire (sometimes silver-plated) or aluminum wire (oxidized) on them. (Fig. 2-1)

Length of commonly used needles: 1.5-2.0 cun (3.75-5.0 centimetres).

Thickness of commonly used needles: No. 28 (0.38 millimetre in diameter).

II. Preparation Before Acupuncture

(1) Selection and Inspection of Needles

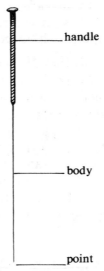

handle

body

point

Fig. 2-1   Structure of an Acupuncture Needle

Prior to applying the needles to the human body, it is imperative to carefully select and inspect the needles to be used. If the needles have loosened handles, or are rusty, or have marks of damage, or are bent and hooked, or have broken tips, discard them.

(2) Repairing and Keeping of Needles

The curved needles can be smoothed out from the handle to the tip repeatedly with the thumb and index finger of one hand while using the other hand to hold the handle.

To protect the needles from being rusted, they should be cleaned with cotton or soft cloth and stored in needle tubes or needle boxes with cotton or gauze cushion to protect the tips from damage due to collision with the hard container.

(3) Practice of Needling

Good needling skills can both reduce the puncture pain and improve the therapeutic effects. Therefore, the practitioners should learn and practice hard to master the needling skills, including the strength of their fingers, the skill to insert and orientate the needle, the coordination of needle manipulation movements, and the skill to twist the needle.

To practise needling skills, a pile of gauze or paper (with cotton flakes put layer by layer between them) may be used first for practice of quick puncture, deep insertion and manipulation of the needle.

(4) Posture of Patient

The patient should be put in a comfortable posture which makes it easy for the physician to accurately locate the stimulating areas and conveniently manipulate the needles. Usually, the sitting posture is selected for scalp acupuncture, but for patients who are extremely weak or with difficulties to sit up, various lying postures can be selected as seen fit by the physician.

(5) Sterilization of Needles and Skin

The needles may be sterilized by autoclave, boiling or soaking in 75 percent alcohol for 20 minutes. The patient's skin where needles will be inserted and the fingers of the physician can be wiped with 75 percent alcohol cotton balls.

III. Manipulation of Acupuncture

From March 1971 through 1972, traditional methods of acupuncture, except the quick manipulation of the needle, were used basically, including rotating insertion of needles obliquely and rotating removal of needles slowly. This technique, apart from its low efficiency, had also the drawback of causing much suffering to the patients. Since 1973, the author of this book began to improve the traditional methods on the basis of repeated clinical practice and summing of experience. And eventually, he has developed the new "three-quickness acupuncture technique," that is, quick insertion, quick manipulation and quick removal of needles. Clinical application shows that the suffering of the patients is reduced and the efficiency is greatly improved.

(1) Insertion of Needles

It contains two steps—prompt puncture into the skin and the quick push of the needle into the deeper layers of tissue.

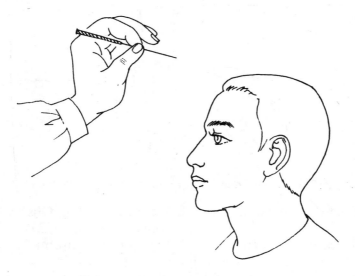

Fig. 2-2   Prompt Puncture into the Skin

1) Prompt puncture: The needle is pinched by the thumb and index finger two centimetres back from the tip. Directed at the targeted stimulating area and with the tips of the thumb and index finger being 5-10 centimetres above the scalp, the tip of the needle is promptly punctured through the skin to the subcutaneous or muscular layer from a distance of 10-20 centimetres (Fig. 2-2) by quickly lifting the back of the hand and pushing down. (Fig. 2-3).

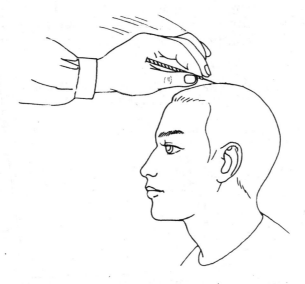

Fig. 2-3   Prompt Puncture into the Skin

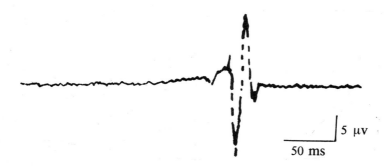

5 μv

50 ms

Fig. 2-4   Electromyogram During Prompt Puncture of the Needle

This method needs only 66 ms to puncture into the skin. Observation method: A Denmark-made 5-μv and 4-channel electromyograph with 50 ms of time base, and 3-cm needle electrode. When the needle electrode was promptly punctured into the forearm, a 40-μv 66-ms wave peak appeared as shown in Fig. 2-4.

On September 26, 1975, a total of 125 patients were made sit in a row for scalp acupuncture treatment at decided stimulating areas. Together, 366 needles were inserted and the time used was only 31 minutes, with the time spent on each patient averaged 14 seconds and the time spent for inserting each needle averaged 5.1 seconds.

By the three-quickness acupuncture method, the manipulation of the needle can be accomplished instantly and the needle is promptly punctured through the skin, so it produces no pain or only slight pain to the patients. On August 4, 1978, the author made a special observation of 337 needle insertions by using a new method to see whether the new method really causes pain to the patients. The results showed that 318 punctures, or 91.1 percent, did not produce any pain at all and 19 punctures, or 8.9 percent, produced slight pain, as shown in Table 2-1.

Table 2-1. Observation of Reflection to Pain Caused by Needling Puncture on August 4-5, 1978

Sensation	Prompt puncture	Quick pushing	Quick twisting	Quick re-moval
Painless	318 (91.1%)	169 (47.5%)	206 (76.0%)	245 (90.1%)
Slight pain	19 (8.9%)	172 (98.3%)	62 (24.0%)	25 (9.9%)
Pain		11 (3.1%)		
Other sensation		4 (1.1%)		
Total	337	359	269	270

2) Quick push: This means, after promptly puncturing needle through the skin, it is quickly pushed inward along the stimulating area to adequate depth without

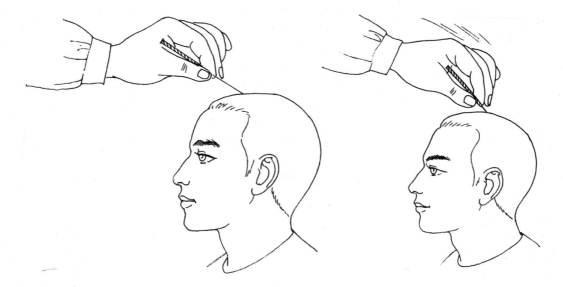

Fig. 2-5   Pushing the Needle Inward with One Hand

the needle being manipulated.

There are two ways to push the needle inward:

(a) Pushing the needle with single hand. Having made the needle puncture through the skin, using the tips of the thumb and index finger to pinch the distal half of the needle (sometimes using the middle finger to touch the tip of needle to make it steady) and push forward along the direction of the stimulating area (Fig. 2-5).

(b) Pushing the needle with two hands. Using the tips of thumb and index finger to pinch the distal half of the needle (with the middle finger in tight touch with the needle) and using the tips of the thumb and index finger of another hand to gently hold the part of the needle close to the scalp (to prevent the needle getting bent during the process of pushing inward), and push the needle forward by both hands (Fig. 2-6).

Pushing the needle inward without manipulation can be used for most patients. But the scalp skin of some patients may be very tough or there is scar in the place where the needle is to be inserted, it is not easy to push the needle inward without manipulation. In such a situation, the needle can be pushed in while manipulating.

Sometimes, the needle may meet a resistance while being pushed inward, this is because the direction or depth of the needle is incorrect or the needle is hindered by the skin or periosteum. In such a situation, the needle should be pulled back a little and pushed forward again after the direction of insertion is adjusted.

(2) Manipulation of Needle

1) Needle-manipulating method

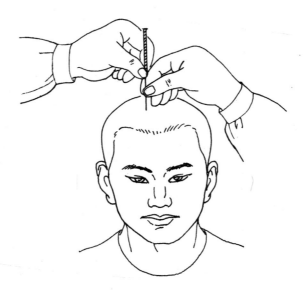

Fig. 2-6   Pushing the Needle Inward with Two Hands

Using the pad of thumb and the radial border of the first joint of the index finger to quickly twist the needle without lifting and thrusting it (Fig. 2-7). While manipulating the needle, the shoulder, elbow, wrist and thumb of the physician must be maintained in a fixed position to avoid changing the direction of the needle.

Normally, the needle is manipulated around 200 times per minute, 405 times

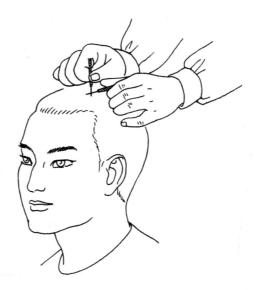

Fig. 2-7   Needle-Manipulating Method

per minute at the most. The manipulation goes on for 0.5-1 minute and then a needling sensation may appear and last for 5-10 minutes. Therefore, the manipulation should be repeated twice after intervals of 5-10 minutes. On August 4-5, 1978, an observation was made on 268 needle insertions with this method, and of them 206, or 76 percent, did not produce any pain, and 62, or 24 percent, produced slight pain.

Quick manipulation of the needle can generate a stronger stimulation in the patient and thus better therapeutic results.

Case Report: Obliterative Disease of the Right Carotid Artery System

Jiang, male, 54 years old, from Yuncheng, Shanxi Province.

Chief complaint: Left hemiplegia for five days.

Case history: On the afternoon of October 17, 1977, the patient suddenly became slurred in speech, developed dripping of saliva and the movement of his left limbs was impaired. The situation continuously deteriorated. Treatment was given with Chinese herbal medicine in a local hospital without any improvement. He was taken in on October 22, 1977.

Past history: Sound health.

Physical examination: The patient had a clear state of mind and normal response. But his speech was slurred. The left eye could not be closed tightly and muscular strength on left side was weak when he was asked to show his teeth. The left arm could raise up only to 120 degrees; the left fingers could extend to 140 degrees (only 90 degrees for the middle finger); there was no gripping strength for the left hand (30 kg for the right hand) while the fingers of the left hand could not touch the palm (leaving a 1-cm gap). The patient had an apparent paralytic gait, although the movement of his left leg appeared to be almost normal. The deep reflexes of his left limbs were exaggerated and the Hoffmann's sign was positive. The pain sensation on left side of body was normal. The blood pressure was 160/100 mmHg.

Diagnosis: Obliterative disease of the right carotid artery system due to hypertension and cerebral arteriosclerosis with left hemiplegia and partial motor aphasia.

Treatment: Applying scalp acupuncture over the right motor area and the motor and sensory area of foot.

Before treatment was given, an electromyogram was made by a Denmark-made four-channel electromyograph with a potential of 200 μv, a time base of 10 ms and a 3-cm needle electrode.

The electrode was inserted to the motor point of left superficial flexor muscle of fingers and then to the motor point of right superficial flexor muscle of fingers.

Observation: The patient was asked to clench both hands, the left hand failed to make into a fist, the gap between the tips of the fingers and the palm was 1 centimetre, and the electromyogram hardly show any electrical discharge. The right hand showed a gripping strength of 30 kg and the electromyogram showed obvious electrical discharge with a peak value of 1 μv (Fig. 2-8).

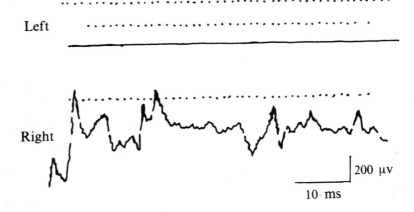

Fig. 2-8   Electromyograms for Both Hands
Before the Needle Was Manipulated

Needling stimulation at the motor area and the motor and sensory area of foot: After the first round of needle manipulation, the gripping strength of left hand increased to 8 kg, and then the electromyogram showed an apparent electrical discharge with a peak value of 1 μv (Fig. 2-9).

After the second round of needle manipulation, the gripping strength of the left hand reached 10 kg and the peak value of electromyogram went up to 1.3 μv (Fig. 2-10).

After the third round of needle manipulation, the gripping strength of the left hand increased again to 14 kg and the peak value of electromyogram further climbed (Fig. 2-11).

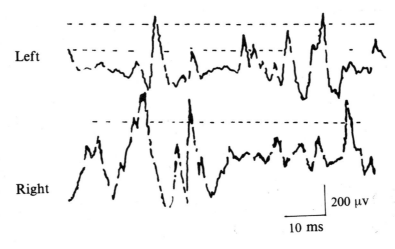

Fig. 2-9   Electromyograms for Both Hands
After the First Round of Needle Manipulation

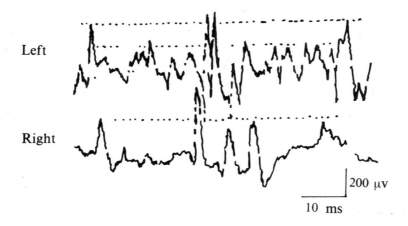

Fig. 2-10   Electromyograms for Both Hands
After the Second Round of Needle Manipulation

Clinical practice over the past 10 years or more shows that manipulating the needles can indeed improve the therapeutic results for some diseases. The bigger the amplitude and the quicker the frequency of the manipulation, the better the therapeutic results.

Now, a machine has been developed to replace the hand in manipulating the needles to treat patients of post-stroke paralysis with satisfactory therapeutic results.

2) Needle-retaining method

The symptoms of some patients are greatly improved or relieved right after the needles are inserted into the stimulating areas. To keep the needles in situs alone

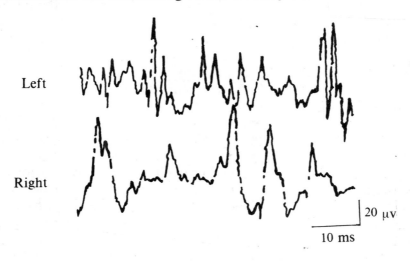

Fig. 2-11   Electromyograms for Both Hands
After the Third Round of Needle Manipulation

for 30 minutes without manipulation could produce a cure effective enough for these patients.

Case Report: Meniere's Syndrome

Wu, male, 40 years old, from Jishan County, Shanxi Province.

Chief complaint: Vertigo and vomiting for one day.

Case history: In early morning that day, the patient suddenly suffered from vertigo and fell down. Turning his head to the right for about 90 degrees, he felt all people and objects rotated, and he had difficulty to turn his head while lying on the left side. So, the patient could not turn his body over and get up from bed. He was admitted on March 3, 1972.

Physical examination: The feeling of rotation of surrounding things was worse when he was asked to turn to the right side. The patient showed a horizontal nystagmus.

Treatment: Immediately after scalp acupuncture was applied at the dizziness and auditory areas on both sides, with the needles being kept in place for 30 minutes, the vertigo disappeared, even when the patient was asked to turn his head to the right, and his vision became clear. After the treatment on the next day, the patient completely recovered and was able to stand up and walk.

For a few patients, there might be some side effects due to manipulating the needles or keeping the needles in place for a long time. For example, a 34-year-old male patient from Kirghizstan came to the author to seek treatment of his headache on July 8, 1992. The neurological examination did not show any positive sign. So, the author inserted needles at the lower two-fifths of the motor and sensory area of foot and sensory area on both sides. After the needles were inserted, he immediately manipulated them for the first round and again 10 minutes later. The needles were made to remain in place 30 minutes. On his visit the next day, the patient complained the aggravation of the headache and general weakness in the afternoon, although the headache was slightly relieved in the morning. Neurological examination again showed a negative sign. In view of the situation, the author improved the treatment by just inserting the needles and made them remain in place for only 10 minutes without manipulation. The headache disappeared after the needles were removed and did not relapse in the afternoon. Since that day, the needles were kept in place for only 10 minutes in each treatment, and a few days later the headache completely gone.

3) Needle-embedding method

There are also some patients whose symptoms and signs showed obvious improvement or even disappeared on the day of treatment by scalp acupuncture. But the symptoms and signs may reappear or become more serious in the same afternoon or on the next day. This may be due to the insufficiency of stimulation. So, the author invented the needle-embedding method to treat these patients. The details of the needle-embedding method are as follows: First, the hair at the stimulating areas where the needles would be inserted is cut and the scalp is sterilized. The needles are inserted and quickly manipulated for three rounds at proper intervals. Then, the needles are not removed but are kept in place for five hours to three days. This method can produce satisfactory therapeutic results in some patients. Yet, if the needles are to remain in place over night, sufficient attention should be given to selecting those needle-insertion points that do not interfere with the patients' sleep and movement.

Case Report:

(1) Obliterative Disease of the Right Carotid Artery System

Jiang, male, 54 years old.

Chief complaint: Partial hemiplegia of left limbs and reduced gripping strength. The patient was admitted on October 22, 1977.

Treatment: Scalp acupuncture was applied at the right motor area and the motor and sensory area of foot. After the first round of needle manipulation, the gripping strength of the left hand increased to 8 kg; after the second round, to 12 kg; and after the third round, to 14 kg. Yet, five hours after the needles were removed, the gripping strength reduced to zero.

Before treatment on October 24, the gripping strength was 7 kg. It increased to 10 kg after the first round of needle manipulation, to 12 kg after the second round, and to 14 kg after the third round. However, it again relapsed to 8 kg five hours after the needles were removed.

The reduction of gripping strength five hours after the removal of needles is due to the insufficiency of stimulation. Hence, the author decided to keep the needles in place for five hours after the three rounds of manipulation stimulation to see if it would be effective.

On October 25, the gripping strength of the patient's left hand was 8 kg before needles were inserted at the right motor area and the motor and sensory area of foot. After the first round of needle manipulation, it increased to 10 kg; after the second round, to 12 kg; and after the third round, to 13 kg. Then, the needles were kept in place for five hours and manipulated again before they were removed. This time the gripping strength did not go down any more. On the contrary, it further increased to 17 kg.

On November 1, the gripping strength of the patient's left hand was 13 kg before treatment. Then, needles were inserted and manipulated for the first round, and the gripping strength increased to 17 kg; after the second round, to 19 kg; and after the third round, it remained at 19 kg. After the needles were kept in place for five hours and removed before one more round of needle manipulation, the gripping strength further went up to 21 kg.

On November 4, before the needles were inserted at the right motor area and the motor and sensory area of foot for treatment, the gripping strength was 19 kg. After the first round of needle manipulation, it remained at 19 kg; and after the second round, it increased to 21 kg; and after the third round, it remained at 21 kg. After keeping the needles in place for five hours before one more round of needle manipulation, the gripping strength increased to 23 kg.

(2) Cervical Spondylosis

Shi, male, 58 years old, from Yuncheng City, Shanxi Province.

Chief complaint: Numbness and pain in the right upper limb for nine months.

Case history: In August 1977, the patient felt mild numbness in his left upper limb without apparent reasons. Since then, the symptom became gradually aggravated. In January 1978, the patient began to feel intermittent attacks of pain once every few minutes while moving the right upper arm forward and backward or trying to raise it. He could not sleep well because of the numbness in the left arm while lying on left side or the pain in the right arm while lying on right side. He tried all sorts of therapies but to not avail. On the contrary, the symptom turned more serious. He could not ride bike and dared not sway his arms while walking for fear of the pain and numbness in the arms. He turned to this hospital for treatment on April 6, 1978.

Physical examination: The patient had a clear state of mind, his speech was normal and no abnormality was found in the cranial nerves. On the lateral side of the left upper arm, a band-shaped area which could help relieve pain by pressing was found; it was 0.5 cm wide. Obvious pain was felt in the deltoid muscle and the lateral side of the clavicle, especially in the forward flexion of the arm. The movement of the right upper limb was limited. His right hand could not reach the pockets in his jacket and his right arm could not be raised up while lying in a deck chair. The head was slightly downward while walking, the elbows were half bent and the upper arms could not move forward and backward. X-ray showed obvious labiate osteophates over the anterior borders of the C3-C7 vertebrae.

Diagnosis: Cervical spondylosis.

Treatment: Scalp acupuncture at the motor and sensory area of foot on both sides; once a day.

First treatment was given on April 6, 1978. After the treatment, the numbness and pain in the arms were relieved, yet reappeared two hours after the needles were removed.

For treatment in the several days that followed, the same situation was observed.

On April 12, the fourth treatment was given. Seven minutes after the needles were inserted, the numbness and pain in the upper limbs disappeared and the movement of the arms turned nimble. Then, the needles were kept in place for 6.5 hours before they were removed. As a result, the symptoms did not relapse in over 24 hours.

The fifth treatment was given on April 14. This time, the needles were embedded in the stimulating areas for 26 hours. The symptoms were all relieved except mild numbness remaining in the left elbow.

4) Needle-removing method

Use the middle or index finger of one hand to slide along the needle down to the scalp (Fig. 2-12) and use the other hand to press a cotton ball over the hole of needle.

In this way, the hair around the hole of the needle can be pushed away and pressed down by the finger.

The handle of the needle may be pinched by the thumb and index finger or by

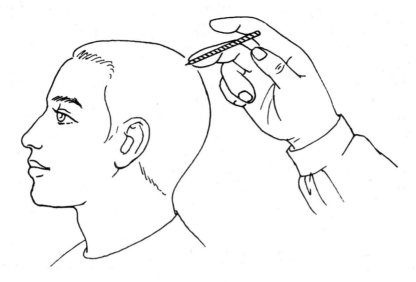

Fig. 2-12   Removal of the Needle

the thumb, index and middle fingers to quickly pull out the scalp (Fig. 2-13).

One-fourth of the needle holes may ooze blood more or less. For those needle holes which ooze one or two drops of blood, the oozing of blood can be stopped by pressing a cotton ball on them for 2-4 seconds. If the hole oozes more blood for 2-3 seconds after the removal of the needle, it should be pressed for 20-40 seconds, or even for one minute to stop the bleeding.

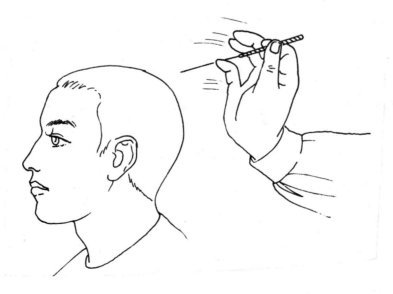

Fig 2-13   Removal of the Needle

Section 2   Observation on Responses to Needling Stimulation

I. Conduction of Common Needling Sensation

(1) Types of Conduction

The common needling conduction includes the hot feeling, numbness and spastic feeling. The hot feeling is very common and may appear in 80 percent of the patients. The original symptoms of numbness, coolness, spastic sensation and pain may be relieved or disappear during the process of scalp acupuncture. Although some patients cannot detect the needling sensation, still the treatment can produce a satisfactory therapeutic result.

(2) Range and Shape of Conduction

(a) For most patients, the conduction reaches the contralateral limbs.

(b) For a small number of patients, the conduction goes to the ipsilateral limbs.

(c) For a tiny few of individuals, the conduction is felt in the whole body.

(d) The conduction is limited to a local area, such as a local joint or a piece of muscle.

(3) Time of Appearance and Disappearance of Needling Sensation

(a) Time of appearance:

It ranges from a few seconds to three minutes in most patients. For a tiny few individuals, it may appear several hours after the needles are removed.

(b) Time to last:

For most patients it lasts for 3-10 minutes. But for a tiny few it may last a few hours and even two days.

II. Band-Shaped Conduction of Needling Sensation

(1) Nature: Hot sensation, numbness, spastic feeling and formication.

(2) Width: 0.5-4.0 centimetres. But in some patients, it may spread over a big patch. To a certain degree, the lasting time is related to the intensity and time of stimulation.

(3) Characteristic of the conductive band: The conductive band may vary in width.

(4) Starting point of conduction: The conduction of needling sensation may start either from the stimulating area, or the nape, or the proximal and middle part of the limbs.

(5) Route of conduction: In most cases, the needling sensation goes from the proximal part to the distal part of the limbs. But in a few cases, it may start from the distal part and go to the proximal part or start from the middle part and spread to both ends.

(6) Relations between the stimulating areas and the range of radiation: Usually, the needling sensation appears either in the limbs of the opposite side or the same side of the stimulating area. In a few patients, it may also appear in parts of the body innervated by the various areas of the cerebral cortex corresponding to the stimulating areas in scalp acupuncture.

(7) Relations between the conductive course of needling sensation and diseases:

According to clinical observation, the conduction of needling sensation may appear both in limbs on the healthy side of the body and limbs on the diseased side. Yet, it is more apparent on the diseased side than on the healthy side. This shows the conduction of needling sensation has some sort of relations with changes in the function of the nervous system caused by the diseases.

(8) Generation of needling sensation and stimulating methods: Usually, the belt-shaped needling sensation is produced by acupuncture. It may also be produced by applying pressure with the handle of the needle, the tip of a pencil and a finger, or moxibustion with a moxa roll. Yet, different stimulating methods may produce needling sensation of different nature.

(9) Simultaneous appearance of a belt of paraesthesia: Application of needling stimulation for 0.5-2 minutes may cause, along the conductive route of the needling sensation, a belt of paraesthesia, characterized by reduced or exaggerated pain sensation, or other modified sensations. Generally speaking, the belt of paraesthesia is wider than the belt-shaped conductive route of the needling sensation, and the abnormal feeling may disappear a few minutes after the stimulation is stopped. But, in some patients it may last for 24 hours.

(10) Characteristic of conduction of needling sensation: The needling sensation may travel along the course of the meridians on the surface of the body and be limited to one limb, and in some cases it may radiate along the topographic distribution of nerve innervation.

(11) Blockage of conduction of needling sensation: In most patients, the conduction of needling sensation can be blocked by injection of procaine or normal saline or by application of pressure. But in some patients it cannot be blocked by any means.

(12) Conductive speed of needling sensation: The quickest is 45 centimetres per second and the slowest is 2.2 centimetres per second, with an average of 10.6 centimetres per second.

(13) Time of disappearance: Usually, the sensation disappears several minutes after the needling stimulation is stopped.

(14) Characteristic of disappearance of needling sensation: In most cases, it disappears at the distal end of the limbs first and the proximal end of the limbs later. But, in some patients it may disappear simultaneously along the whole route of conduction.

III. Involuntary Movement, a Response to
Needling Stimulation

(1) Involuntary Movement of Limbs

(a) The diseased limbs may be lifted up involuntarily and the arms may even be raised up over the head, during needling stimulation.

(b) The limbs may move involuntarily during needling stimulation.

(c) The paralytic limbs may automatically extend and stretch, in some cases exceeding the normal range during needling stimulation.

(d) Some paralytic patients may involuntarily stand up and even walk around during needling stimulation.

(e) The diseased limbs may jerk spasmodically during needling stimulation.

(2) Automatic Movement of Internal Organs

(a) The patients may cough spontaneously or continuously during needling stimulation.

2) In a few patients, the intensity of peristalsis of the stomach and intestines may increase apparently.

IV. Perspiration in Face and Limbs

In a few cases, the patients may have sweat in the contralateral (or ipsilateral occasionally) side of the face and palm; sometimes the sweat may even drop down.

V. Apparent Improvement of Physical Symptoms

For about 10 percent of the paralytic patients, the first round of scalp acupuncture treatment may produce an apparent improvement of their physical symptoms of paralysis.

VI. Temporary Exacerbation of Physical Symptoms

A temporary exacerbation of the physical symptoms may be witnessed in some patients during needling stimulation. But this phenomenon will usually disappear a few minutes after the needles are removed, although it may last several hours in a tiny number of patients. After this spell, a general improvement will be achieved in the patients' physical symptoms.

Case Report:

(1) Exacerbated Soreness and Weakness of Limbs and Fever After Needling Stimulation

Zhang, male, 72 years old, from Yuncheng, Shanxi Province.

Chief complaint: Hemiplegia of right limbs for 18 days.

Case history: The patient suddenly developed hemiplegia in the right limbs 18 days before without losing consciousness.

Physical examination: The patient had a clear state of mind and could speak normally. Examination proved that his tongue deviated slightly to the right side and his right arm and leg were completely paralysed.

Treatment: After three rounds of scalp acupuncture at the upper three-fifths of the motor area and the motor and sensory area of foot on the left side, much improvement was witnessed in the paralysis and reduction of muscular strength of the right limbs, which could not only move normally but also have certain muscular strength. Yet, the right hand still suffered from numbness.

On January 15, 1978, acupuncture was given to the upper three-fifths of the motor area and middle two-fifths of the sensory area on the left side. When the needles were inserted, the patient felt hotness in the right shoulder, which spread along the arm to the hand three minutes later and then to the right lower limb five minutes later. The soreness, discomfort and weakness of the right arm and hand thus caused lasted for more than 10 hours. On the next day, however, the patient felt much relaxed. The same phenomenon was repeatedly observed after scalp acupuncture treatment in three successive days. An examination on January 18 verified that the numbness of the hand had gone, the gripping strength of both hands increased to 28 kg and the Barre's sign was negative. Again, needles were inserted at the middle two-fifths of the sensory area as well as upper three-fifths of the motor area and the motor and sensory area of foot on the left side without needle manipulation. Two minutes later hotness was felt in the right shoulder, and five minutes later hotness and soreness were felt in the right fingers. The gripping strength of the left hand was still 28 kg, while that of the right hand went down to 18 kg. Five minutes after the removal of the needles, the hot feeling of the right fingers gradually reduced. And 10 minutes after the removal of the needles, the patient still felt some hotness in the right fingers. Then, the movement of the hand was more nimble than before the treatment and the gripping strength of the right hand increased to 26 kg.

(2) Exacerbated Pain in Leg During Needling Stimulation

Zong, male, 20 years old, from Yuncheng, Shanxi Province.

Chief complaint: Pain in left leg for six months.

Case history: Six months before, the patient developed without any particular reason lumbago, which was followed by pain on the lateral aspect of the left leg, and treatment with medicinal herbs and by common acupuncture failed to produce any therapeutic effect. He went to the author for help on January 16, 1978 and physical examination verified pain in the waist and left leg accompanied with cough and tenderness in the popliteal fossa when asked to bend down.

Diagnosis: Neuralgia sciatica on the left side.

Treatment: Applying scalp acupuncture at the upper two-fifths of the right motor area and right motor and sensory area of foot. Two minutes after the needles were inserted, the pain in the left leg became more serious. Two hours after the needles were removed, the feeling of exaggerated pain in the leg disappeared. Then the patient felt that the pain in his left lower limb was much relieved. The same phenomenon of feeling exacerbated pain in the left leg occurred each time in all the follow-up five rounds of scalp treatment, yet after each round of treatment general improvement was witnessed.

VII. Syncope During Acupuncture Treatment

During acupuncture treatment, if the patients suddenly develop a spell of repeated yawning and their facial complexion changes, this is a premonitory sign of syncope. If syncope really occurs, the patient may show such manifestations as pale complexion, chest distress, palpitation, dizziness, blurred vision, nausea, profuse perspiration and cold limbs.

Prevention: For first-visit patients, they should be asked whether they have had fainting spells in acupuncture treatment and less intensive stimulation should be given to patients who have weak physique and who are nervous, hungry and tired.

The method to deal with the situation: Needling syncope is due to temporary cerebral ischemia. To cope with the situation, the needles should be immediately removed and the patients are lain down and are given some hot water to drink, or cover their foreheads with towels wetted with hot water. In normal conditions, the needling syncope can be relieved in several minutes.

To deal with needling does not mean to discontinue scalp acupuncture treatment for patients who faint during treatment or have the history of syncope. It only means to adopt a method to deal with the needling syncope first and then continue the treatment.

There are two ways to prevent needling syncope:

(1) Reducing stimulating intensity

For patients who have fainting spells when stimulating intensity is increased by manipulating the needles in previous treatment, the needle-manipulating method should be avoided and replaced by the needle-retaining method in later treatment. Clinical practice proves that this can also produce quite satisfactory therapeutic results.

Case Report: Syncope During Needling Stimulation

Hou, female, 53 years old, from Yuncheng, Shanxi Province.

Chief complaint: Left hemiplegia for 11 days.

Case history: On July 14, 1978, the patient suddenly contracted headache and developed numbness and poor mobility in the left limbs when she was working in the field. When she was carried home, her left leg was completely paralysed. As treatment with both Western and traditional Chinese medicine had failed to produce a satisfactory cure, she was brought to the author for treatment.

Physical examination: The patient had a clear state of mind and could speak normally. She would fall back down if made to sit by herself and her left foot could not be lifted up when she was asked to walk with others' support. Her left arm was too weak to hold a bowl and to do any delicate things.

Diagnosis: Cerebral thrombosis of right anterior cerebral artery.

Treatment: Scalp acupuncture was applied at the upper three-fifths of the right motor area and right motor and sensory area of foot. When the needles were promptly punctured into the scalp, the patient did not give any abnormal responses. When the needles were manipulated to intensify the stimulation several minutes later, the patient suddenly developed dizziness, blurred vision, vexation and cool limbs. The needles were immediately removed and the symptoms gradually disappeared in a few minutes. In the treatment the next day, the needles were merely inserted and kept in place for 30 minutes without needle manipulation, and no needling syncope developed and the patient's muscular strength was slightly improved. After five rounds of treatment, the muscular strength of her left arm was greatly improved and the movement of her left hand became much more flexible to hold things; her left leg became stronger and the patient could walk by herself. The hemiplegia was basically cured after 12 rounds of treatment.

(2) Gradual Increase of Stimulating Intensity

For patients with history of needling syncope, the initial stimulation should be very gentle and the stimulating intensity should be gradually increased to let the patients gradually adapt to the needling stimulation. Usually, the stimulation should be increased in three steps: Immediately removing needles, keeping needles in place for some time and manipulating needles.

Case Report: Hemiplegia on the Right Side

Xie, male, 53 years old, from Hebei Province.

Chief complaint: Hemiplegia on the right side accompanied with numbness in the left side of the head and dizziness for five years.

Case history: On December 10, 1977, the patient suddenly developed dizziness and inhibited mobility of the right limbs accompanied by difficulty in walk when he was travelling by train. He also had numbness in the left limbs and slurred speech. Treatment by Western and traditional Chinese medicine did not produce any satisfactory results. He was admitted on August 26, 1978.

Physical examination: The patient had a clear state of mind but could not speak clearly. When he was asked to point his nose with his right hand, he could not point at the right place. He deviated to the right while walking. Therefore, he needed a walking stick to support his body while standing and walking. The sensation of pain on the left side of his body was reduced.

Diagnosis: Cerebral arteriosclerosis with thrombosis of posterior inferior cerebellar artery.

Treatment: Scalp acupuncture was applied at the balance areas on both sides on August 26, 1978. When the needles were manipulated for the first round 10 minutes after they were inserted, the patient suddenly developed a pale complexion, profuse perspiration, blurred vision and vexation. In view of this situation, the needles were immediately removed and the patient was made to lie flat to rest. Half an hour later, the symptoms of needling syncope disappeared entirely. The physical signs were normal. On the next day, the needles were inserted into the balance areas on both sides and then removed instantly, and there were no unfavourable reactions. When treatment was given for the fourth time, the needles were kept in place 30 minutes, still no unfavourable reactions. In the fifth round of treatment, the needles were not only manipulated but also kept in place for as long as two hours. The patient did not develop needling syncope. Rather, his limbs became more nimble and he could walk more stably.

VIII. Unfavourable Reactions During and
After Scalp Acupuncture

Scalp acupuncture is generally save and does not produce any bad effects in most patients. Yet, it may give rise to some unfavourable reactions in a small number of patients, which include local pain, toothache or itching over the head during treatment, and the palpitation, shortness of breath, general discomfort, fever and edema after treatment. Most of these reactions will disappear a few seconds to several minutes after the needles are removed. But, edema may last several days. Generally speaking, it is not necessary to give special treatment to these symptoms. For a tiny number of patients who show strong unfavourable reactions and in whom the therapy seems to fail to produce apparent cure, scalp acupuncture may be temporarily discontinued.

Case Report:

(1) Itching in Head Vertex When Scalp Acupuncture Was Applied at Motor and Sensory Area of Foot and Upper Two-Fifths of Sensory Area

Cui, female, 46 years old, from Luoyang, Henan Province.

Chief complaint: General arthralgia for nine months.

Case history: The patient developed numbness of the left arm and arthralgia all over the body without any apparent cause nine months before. She was admitted to the hospital on September 12, 1978.

Physical examination: The patient had a clear state of mind and spoke clearly; there were no positive neurological signs, no deformity of the joints and no itching in the head.

Treatment: Scalp acupuncture was applied at the motor and sensory areas of foot and the upper two-fifths of the sensory areas on both sides. Shortly after the needles were inserted, the patient felt itching and formication over in the centre of the head vertex, which quickly spread to the parietal tubers on both sides, the area between eyebrows and the area over the parieto-occipital sutures. The itching sensation disappeared one hour after the needles were removed. The same phenomenon was observed during all six rounds of treatment.

(2) Toothache Due to Scalp Acupuncture at Lower Two-Fifths of Sensory Area

Kang, female, 37 years old.

Chief complaint: Insomnia for more than three years.

Case history: The patient began to suffer from insomnia three years before and headache recently.

Treatment: Scalp acupuncture was applied at the upper two-fifths and lower two-fifths of the sensory area on both sides. When a needle was inserted at the lower two-fifths of the sensory area, the patient felt spastic pain radiated from the needle point through the preauricular region to the molar teeth for more than half an hour. The pain was particularly serious when she tried to turn her head to the left. When the needle was pulled out to the subcutaneous layer and again inserted along the muscular layer, the pain disappeared.

(3) Left Ear Tinnitus Caused by Scalp Acupuncture at Motor and Sensory Area of Foot

Liu, male, 68 years old, Yuncheng, Shanxi Province.

Chief complaint: Hemiplegia of left limbs for more than one year.

Treatment: On October 13, 1978, scalp acupuncture was applied at the upper three-fifths of the right motor area and the motor and sensory area of foot. After the needles punctured the flesh, the patient felt a windy noise in his left ear for 20 minutes.

(4) Edema of Right Leg Caused by Scalp Acupuncture at Upper Two-Fifths of Left Motor Area

Liu, male, 68 years old, from Yuncheng, Shanxi Province.

Chief complaint: Hemiplegia of left limbs for more than one year.

Case history: On May 3, 1977, the patient suddenly developed left hemiplegia while working in the field, without losing consciousness. The patient was admitted September 9, 1978.

Physical examination: The patient had a clear state of mind and could speak normally. His left nasolabial groove was a bit shallow and his tongue deviated to the left while protruding. His left arm could only be raised up to the level of the shoulder, and his left hand could bent but not stretch. The left leg was weak and he had an apparent hemiplegic gait to walk with the right toes sliding over the floor.

Diagnosis: Chronic cerebral thrombosis with hemiplegia of left limbs.

Treatment: Scalp acupuncture treatment was given at the right motor and sensory area of foot and the upper three-fifths of the motor area. After five rounds of treatment, the patient could extend his left hand normally and walk steadily. During the sixth round of treatment, scalp acupuncture was also applied at the upper two-fifths of the motor area on the left side for observation of the needling sensation. Next day after the treatment, the patient developed a pitting edema over the right tibia bone and the dorsum of the right foot.

(5) General Edema Caused by Scalp Acupuncture at Motor and Sensory Area of Foot and Upper Two-Fifths of Motor Area on Both Sides

Huang, female, 18 years old, from Yuncheng, Shanxi Province.

Chief complaint: Paralysis of both legs for 16 years.

Case history: The patient's legs were paralysed 16 years before after an attack of high fever. She could not stand and walk because of the apparent amyotrophy. She was admitted to the hospital on June 17, 1978.

Physical examination: The patient could not stand and walk due to paralysis of both legs, so she could only move with the support of a stool. Both her legs were atrophic and the circumference of bilateral gastrocnemius muscles as the thickest part of the leg was only 24 cm. The skin was cool, but not swollen and the sensation of the skin was normal.

Diagnosis: Sequelae of poliomyelitis.

Treatment: Scalp acupuncture was applied at the motor and sensory area of foot and the upper two-fifths of the motor area on both sides once a day. After the first treatment, the patient felt distended in the legs. After the third round of treatment, she developed a slight edema in the both legs, which became increasingly more obvious and pitting in nature. The patient had also felt numbness in the legs and a hot sensation when she tried to walk. The heart beat was normal and valvular murmur was absent. She felt no knocking pain over the kidney and no frequent, urgent and painful urination, and the routine examination of urine was normal. The edema remained through to the tenth round of treatment. But, the pitting edema over the tibia bone completely disappeared when the treatment was stopped for eight days. Then, after three additional rounds of treatment were given, edema of the eyelids and face and pitting edema of the legs reappeared. Examination verified that the heart and lungs remained normal and the blood pressure was 120/80 mmHg. There was no frequent and urgent urination. The test of urine was also normal.

(6) Fever and General Hot Sensation Caused by Scalp Acupuncture at Sensory Area

Ma, male, 25 years old, from Yuncheng, Shanxi Province.

Chief complaint: Dizziness and poor memory for several years.

Case history: The patient suffered a trauma in the head when he was four years old. Since then, he felt dizziness and his memory was impaired. Treatment by both Western and traditional Chinese medicine effected little cure. He turned to the hospital for help on August 8, 1978.

Physical examination: The patient had a clear state of mind and could normally express himself. There were no positive signs for the neurological system.

Treatment: Scalp acupuncture was applied at the upper two-fifths and lower two-fifths of the sensory area on both sides. Next morning after the first round of treatment, the patient developed general fever, discomfort, weakness and soreness in the whole body, yet without nasal obstruction and running nose. The same phenomenon was repeatedly observed in all five rounds of treatment. The body temperature before each round of treatment was 37.1 degrees (subaxillary) and the routine blood examination and eosinophil leucocyte count were normal. After the sixth round of treatment, the patient still had fever and general malaise up until 3 p.m. The body temperature was 37.5 degrees. But, the routine blood examination and eosinophil cell count still remained normal.

IX. Prevention and Handling of Unexpected Conditions

(1) Bending of Needle

The needles used in acupuncture treatment may be bent inside or outside the skin of the patient. But, in scalp acupuncture this situation happens only outside the scalp due to poor manipulation of the needles. If this situation happens, the bent needle should be removed from the scalp and a new needle should be used to continue the treatment.

(2) Stuck of Needle

If the needles cannot be manipulated in the tissue or easily pulled out from the body, this is called the stuck of needle. Such a situation is usually caused by muscular tension or muscular spasm. In this situation, the stuck needle can be removed by gentle manipulation.

X. Course of Treatment

For chronic diseases, such paralysis, one course of treatment usually lasts 10 to 12 days. The second course should follow after an interval of 3-5 days.

XI. Other Methods of Stimulation

(1) Plum-Blossom Acupuncture

After the needle and the therapeutic area over the skin are sterilized, use one hand to hold the handle of the plum-blossom needle to tap repeatedly and rhythmically at the stimulating area with proper pressure applied by moving the index finger until the skin of the stimulating area turns flushed and congested.

(2) Moxibustion: Moxa rolls are often used. First select the right stimulating area and cut the hair, then light the tip of a moxa roll and hold it 1.5 centimetres over the selected stimulating area to produce a hot sensation. This process lasts for about 20-30 minutes. The distance between the scalp and the tip of the moxa roll can be appropriately adjusted according to the tolerance of the patients. This method is usually used to treat extremely weak patients.

(3) Acupressure: This method is used when needles and moxa rolls are not available. It means to select the right stimulating area or areas to use the thumb to press or knead it repeatedly.

All three methods can produce some treatment for certain diseases.

Section 3 Observation on the Law of Appearance of Needling Sensation

In clinical practice of scalp acupuncture, it has been discovered that needle manipulating stimulation can always induce a needling sensation in the limbs to produce a better therapeutic effect in the patients. But, just inserting the needles in place and keep them there for 30 minutes without twisting them to produce the needling sensation can also relieve the symptoms in some patients.

I. Range of Observation

The observation was made on 203 patients with eight kinds of diseases, including the cerebral thrombosis with sequelae, cerebral haemorrhage with sequelae, and cerebral arteriosclerosis with insufficiency of blood supply. All these selected patients had a clear state of mind and could respond normally to inquiries.

II. Methods of Observation

(1) Observation of Appearance of Needling Sensation After Insertion of Needle

Needles were inserted at the six stimulating areas separately, and observations were made in each case on the radiating range and duration of the needling sensation (hotness, numbness or twitching sensation).

(2) Observation on Appearance of Needling Sensation Produced by Different Stimulating Methods

To study the impact of different stimulating methods (the insertion of needle, manipulating the needle twice, lifting and thrusting the needle once, and tapping the handle of the needle once) on the needling sensation—time of appearance and disappearance of the needling sensation as well as its radiating range, we selected six patients (Table 2-2). Careful observation proved that all different methods of stimulation could produce needling sensation in all six patients. The only difference was in the radiating range of the needling sensation.

**Table 2-2. Comparison of Appearance of
Needling Sensation Caused by Different Stimulations**

Subject	Stimulation	Time of appearance (minute)	Time of persistence (minute)	Location and nature of needling sensation
Chen with Parkinsonism	Insertion of needle	4	37	Hotness in left hand and leg
	Twisting 2 turns	12	7	ditto
	One lifting and thrusting of needle	2	24	ditto
	One tapping at the handle of needle	5.5	19	ditto
Li with cerebral thrombosis	Insertion of needle	3	39	Hotness in left palm and leg
	Twisting 2 turns	5	2	Hotness in chest, back & left leg
	One lifting and thrusting of needle	7	29	ditto
	One tapping at the handle of needle	2	8	ditto
Qiao with cerebral thrombosis	Insertion of needle	30 sec.	34	Hotness in left arm and leg
	Twisting 2 turns	7	13	Hotness in left leg
	One lifting and thrusting of needle	2.5	29	ditto
	One tapping at the handle of needle	40 sec.	21	ditto
Liang with cerebral thrombosis	Insertion of needle	3	29	Hotness in head, right arm & leg
	Twisting 2 turns	2.5	11	Hotness in right arm & leg
	One lifting and thrusting of needle	2	7	Hotness in head, right arm & leg
	One tapping at the handle of needle	2	8	Hotness in right arm & leg
Gao with cerebral thrombosis	Insertion of needle	2	34	Hotness in chest back & left leg, twitch of fingers of 2 hands
	Twisting 2 turns	10 sec.	7	Hotness in chest, back & right leg
	One lifting and thrusting	2.33	8	ditto
	One tapping at handle	2	8	ditto

Case Report: Change of Location of Needling Sensation After Manipulating the Needle

Wu, male, 69 years old, from Jishan County, Shanxi Province.

Chief complaint: Cerebral arteriosclerosis and insufficient blood supply to the plain.

Treatment: Scalp acupuncture applied at the upper two-fifths of the left sensory area.

Observation: The treatment was given on August 12, 1972. When a needle was inserted into the upper two-fifths of the left sensory area (1 cm beside the median line), the patient felt a hot sensation spreading backward, in the shape of a belt of 0.5 centimetre, along the median line to the neck and then downward along the posterior median line of the back to the Changqiang (GV 1) acupoint. The duration was two minutes. When the needle was again manipulated for 1.5 minutes, the patient felt instant dizziness in the head and numbness, also a belt 0.5 cm wide, spreading from the posterior and distal border of the axillary fossa along the posteriolateral border of the right upper limb to the wrist. The duration was 4 minutes.

In both cases, the duration of the needling sensation produced by the insertion of needle was longer than that caused by any other stimulating method (Table 2-2).

(3) Observation of Relations Between Duration of Needling Sensation and Different Types of Stimulation

Five patients were chosen to study respectively the duration of needling sensation caused by the insertion of needle, the manipulation of needle for two seconds and the manipulation of needle for 20-30 minutes. The observation proved that the needling sensation was caused in all five patients by the insertion of needle and, moreover, the sensation could reappear when the needle was manipulated. But, the duration of needling sensation caused by the insertion of needle was much longer than that produced by needle manipulation. In any case, the duration of the needling sensation was within 30 minutes. The observation also proved that continued manipulation of needle for 20-30 minutes could not produce more lasting needling sensation, which usually disappeared before the needle manipulation was stopped (Figs. 2-6, 2-7 and 2-8).

(4) Observation on Cases in Which Needling Sensation Was Absent

Fifteen patients with cerebrovascular diseases were selected for this study. All the 15 patients did not feel the needling sensation within 30 minutes after needles were inserted. The study also found that no needling was produced when the needles were manipulated for 30 minutes.

In acupuncture applied to the body, it is generally stressed to use the manipulation, lifting and thrusting of the needles to promote the obtaining of qi (deqi). But, in the practice of scalp acupuncture, it has been found the insertion of the needle itself can generate a needling sensation, or, in other words, cause the obtaining of qi.

For most patients who can feel the needling sensation when needles are just inserted, needle manipulation, lifting and thrusting as well as tapping of the needle handle can also be used to bring the needling sensation to reappear. This testifies that the needling sensation can be produced again in patients who feel it when the needles are just inserted.

For those patients in whom the insertion of needle produces a needling sensation, manipulation of the needle for 20-30 minutes can also make it reappear. Yet, the needling sensation usually disappear before the needle manipulation stops. This means the lengthening of the time to manipulate the needle does not necessarily lengthen the duration of the needling sensation.

For patients in whom the needling sensation does not appear in 30 minutes after the insertion of needle, manipulating the needles for 30 minutes will not make it appear either. This shows that in scalp acupuncture the manipulation of the needle can only produce a needling sensation in those patients who feel the sensation when the needle is inserted, but not in those who do not feel the sensation at the time when the needle is inserted.

Section 4   Observation of Changes in Body Temperature in Patients Who Feel Hot During Acupuncture Treatment

I. Observation of Changes in Body Temperature in Patients Feeling a Hot Sensation During Scalp Acupuncture Treatment

About 80 percent of patients receiving scalp acupuncture treatment can feel a hot needling sensation. In order to study whether the hot feeling caused by scalp acupuncture would lead to a change of the local body temperature, a semiconductor thermometer was used to measure the local temperature changes of 16 patients before, during and after the scalp acupuncture.

Among the 16 patients, seven felt the hot needling sensation, all accompanied by a rise of body temperature in places where the hot needling sensation was most conspicuously felt, with the most remarkable rise being 2.4 degrees centigrade; four had a numbness spasmodic sensation; and five did not feel anything and the local body temperature remained unchanged.

Case Report:

(1) Peng, male, 34 years old, from Kedong County, Heilongjiang Province.

The patient had suffered from mild hemiplegia and numbness on the right side of the body for seven months and went to the hospital for treatment on December 3, 1974. He basically recovered after scalp acupuncture treatment. During the treatment, the patient often felt hot in his right palm when needles were inserted at the upper three-fifths of the left motor area.

On December 24, 1974, the patient again felt a hot sensation in his right palm. The semiconductor thermometer was used to record the local temperature difference before and after the treatment.

(a) Before treatment, the temperature of both palms was 6.8 degrees centigrade.

(b) During treatment, a hot needling sensation was felt in the right palm and the local skin temperature increased to 8.8 degrees, while the skin temperature of the left palm remained unchanged at 6.8 degrees.

(c) One hour after the needle was removed, the patient felt the hot feeling in the right palm had come down. Measurement by the semiconductor showed that the skin temperature of the right palm changed to 4.5 degrees, while that of the left palm was 5 degrees.

(2) Bai, male, 34 years old

The patient had suffered from hemiplegia in the right of the body for more than one year. On August 4, 1975, he was admitted to the hospital for treatment by scalp acupuncture applied at the left motor and sensory area of foot. Like in the previous case, the semiconductor thermometer was used to observe his body temperature changes. Before treatment, the skin temperature at his right sole was 3.6 degrees.

(a) When the needle was retained in place for 12 minutes, the patient felt a slight hot sensation in his right sole. At this time, the temperature there went up to 4.6 degrees.

(b) When the needle was kept in place for 35 minutes, the temperature remained at 4.6 degrees.

(c) When the needle was kept in place for 48 minutes, the patient felt the hot sensation radiated to the right leg, the thermometer showed that the skin temperature at the right sole increased to 5.1 degrees.

(d) when the needle was retained for one and half hours, the patient felt the hot sensation in the right sole somewhat came down, and the thermometer indicated the local temperature at the right sole decreased to 4.4 degrees.

(e) After the needle was retained for two hours, the patient felt the hot sensation at the right sole completely disappeared. As a result, the local temperature further went down to 4 degrees.

II. Observation on Changes in Body Temperature
in Patients Feeling a General Hot
Needling Sensation

The needle-embetting method of scalp acupuncture may produce a general hot feeling in a tiny number of patients, because of which there may also appear an apparent rise of body temperature. The subjective feverish feeling and the objective change of body temperature would both disappear after the needles are removed.

Case Report:

Cai, male, 37 years old.

Chief complaint: Headache for two years. The headache often concentrate at temporal region on both sides and occasionally in the frontal and occipital regions. The headache was often accompanied by irritation and impaired vision, with the visual acuity being 0.4 for the left eye and 0.5 for the right eye. The headache was improved by the treatment with scalp acupuncture.

Physical examination: The tongue deviated to the right when protruded and fundiscopic examination did not found edema at the optic disc.

Treatment: when needles were embedded in the scalp for eight hours, the patient would have a general feverishness feeling similar to that which was observed in common cold. As such time, body temperature would increase to 38 degrees (subaxillary). Ten minutes after the needles were removed, it would return to normal. The same phenomenon was observed in all four rounds of treatment. Each time when the patient had a general feverish feeling, there would be simultaneous general perspiration.

Summary

The above study proves that both general and local hot feeling caused by scalp acupuncture are accompanied by an increase of local skin temperature or body temperature, and whenever the hot feeling goes, the body temperature will return to normal. This indicates that scalp acupuncture can produce both a subjective hot sensation and an objective increase of body temperature.

Section 5 Aqueous Acupuncture and Acupressure

Besides acupuncture, other stimulating methods can also be applied to the stimulating areas over the scalp to treat diseases.

I. Aqueous Acupuncture at Stimulating Areas

It has been proved to be a fairly effective method to treat cerebral dysgenesis by injecting 250 mg of N-acetylglutamic acid and 20 mg of furathiamine into the motor area, the mento-emotional area and the first, second and third speech areas together with a hot compress to promote their absorption once a day or once every two days. Altogether, 50 cases of cerebral dysgenesis have been treated with this method, 37 (or 74 percent) obtained apparent therapeutic results and 7 (or 14 percent) obtained certain therapeutic effect. This indicates that aqueous acupuncture applied at the stimulating areas over the scalp is effective to treat cerebral diseases.

II. Acupressure at Stimulating Areas

Acupressure applied over the reproductive area and intestinal area on both sides can be used to treat functional uterine bleeding, prolapse of uterus, irregular menstruation, dysmenorrhoea and diseases of the nervous system. This method has been used to treat 136 patients with the above-mentioned disorders. It has cured 88 (or 64.7 percent) of them, has brought improvement to 46 (33.9 percent), and has proved to be ineffective in 2 (1.4 percent). The acupressure, if applied at the tender areas or areas that are more sensitive to pain, will produce a better result.

CHAPTER 3
CLINICAL PRACTICE

Scalp acupuncture has been practised for more than 20 years since 1970. Extensive clinical practice of physicians both at home and abroad has indicated that scalp acupuncture can be applied to treat more than 100 diseases, and it is particularly effective in treating diseases due to pathological lesions in the brain and diseases of the internal organs that are related to the dysfunction of the cerebral cortex.

Section 1 Diseases of Nervous System

I. Cerebrovascular Diseases

Cerebrovascular diseases are common disorders that endanger the health and life of human beings. Scalp acupuncture applied at the motor area and sensory area can bring a market improvement to or even completely cure 70 percent of patients with such diseases. Moreover, scalp acupuncture has the advantage of being effectiveness, economical, simple and safe. Therefore, it is one of the best therapeutic methods to treat cerebrovascular diseases.

Besides causing high mortality, cerebrovascular diseases often cause paralysis and other serious sequelae, and so they are diseases that bring serious harm to the health of human beings.

China has a long history and accumulated rich experiences in preventing and treating cerebrovascular diseases. *Internal Canon of the Yellow Emperor*, which was compiled as early as the Spring and Autumn and Warring States periods, recorded in great detail methods to treat cerebrovascular diseases with medicinal herbs and acupuncture. In modern Western medicine, there are also many drugs and methods which have been proved effective in treating cerebrovascular diseases.

Yet, treatment with medicinal herbs, acupuncture and Western drugs can only provide a fundamental cure to or improve the symptoms of one-fourth to one-third of the patients of cerebrovascular diseases. Therefore, to actively prevent and treat cerebrovascular diseases is of great importance to the health of the people.

According to our statistics collected over a period of 22 years since 1970, however, of the total of 32,332 cases treated with scalp acupuncture, there were 20,923 cases of cerebrovascular diseases, accounting for 64.7 percent. Of the 20,923 cases of cerebrovascular diseases, 7,637 were cured, accounting for 36.5 percent; 7,117 witnessed marked improvement in their symptoms, accounting for 34.0 percent; and another 5,196 witnessed lesser degrees of improvement, accounting for 24.8 percent.

Therefore, with its advantage of being highly effective, economical and safe, scalp acupuncture can be considered a good therapy for cerebrovascular diseases.

(1) Cerebral Thrombosis

The pathological lesions in the cerebral blood vessels, such as atherosclerosis, are the primary pathogenetic factor for cerebral thrombosis, while the increase of coagulation of blood and the reduction of blood flow are considered as secondary factors. The onset of diseases may be either slow or prompt, and in some cases there are prodromal symptoms, such as headache and dizziness. As the lesions occur at different locations, the clinical symptoms of the disease are also different. For example, the lesion in the cortical branch of the middle cerebral artery may cause hemiplegia of the contralateral limbs, with the upper limb more badly attacked or completely paralysed. The recovery of such paralysis usually starts from the lower limb while the upper limb remains either permanently paralysed or semi-paralysed. Thrombosis in the anterior cerebral artery may also paralysis that is more severe in the lower limb than in the upper limb, whose recovery usually starts from the upper limb while the lower limb witnesses a much later and slower improvement or remains paralysed permanently. As the cerebral lesions may occur in different small branches of the cortical cortex, other different clinical symptoms, such as aphasia, abnormal sensation and apraxia, may also appear.

In addition, the severity of the clinical symptoms is often not in proportion with the size of the artery involved and the degree of obstruction in the artery. For example, complete obstruction of the internal carotid artery by thrombosis at its original part may only cause partial impairment of the function of the hands, whereas the thrombosis at the cortical branch of the middle cerebral artery may cause complete paralysis of the upper limbs. This phenomenon may be related to the compensation of collateral blood circulation. In some patients with marked paralysis, the arteriogram cannot show any defect of the contrast medium in the blood vessel.

Selected stimulating areas: The motor area, sensory area and motor and sensory area of foot on the contralateral side of the physical symptoms.

Treatment: After the diagnosis is confirmed and the acute symptoms are brought under control, scalp acupuncture should be applied as early as possible. The therapeutic result is evidently related to the course of the disease. In general, the shorter the course of the disease, the better the therapeutic result. Nevertheless, a marked improvement can also be achieved in some chronic cases.

The therapeutic result is also related to the location of the lesion. Scalp acupuncture produces a better therapeutic result for patients with thrombosis in the branches of the middle and anterior cerebral arteries and a poorer therapeutic result in patients with thrombosis in the main trunk and deeper branches of the artery.

In addition, the therapeutic result is related to the functions of the cerebral cortex and the compensation of collateral blood circulation.

In some cases, the prodromal symptoms may last a long time. If they can be discovered and treated at an earlier time, the condition can be brought under control and its deterioration be prevented.

Of the 6,630 cases of cerebral thrombosis treated with scalp acupuncture, 2,524 cases, or 37.88 percent of the total, were basically cured; 2,145 cases, or 32.19 percent, were noticeably relieved; 1,733 cases, or 26 percent, witnessed some improvement; 259 cases, or 3.8 percent, did no show any improvement; and 2 cases, or 0.03 percent, deteriorated. This proves that scalp acupuncture can produce a good therapeutic effect in the treatment of cerebral thrombosis.

The following is a summary of the various factors affecting the therapeutic effect of scalp acupuncture on the basis of clinical experience gained over 22 years.

(a) Case History and Therapeutic Effect

As early as in 1971, the author of this book and his colleagues found that there was a close relationship between the therapeutic effect of scalp acupuncture and the case history of cerebral thrombosis, that is, the shorter the case history, the better the therapeutic result can scalp acupuncture achieve. In order to make the study convenient, they divided 500 patients of cerebral thrombosis into two groups —the 304 patients with a case history of less than three months were made as one group and the 196 patients with a case history of longer than three months were made as another group. Of the former group, 145 patients were basically cured, accounting for 47.80 percent. But only 45 patients of the second group were basically cured, accounting for 23 percent. The difference in cure rate was significant.

Why is the shorter case history so important to satisfactory therapeutic result? This is because at the early stage of cerebral thrombosis, the damage of the brain tissue around the blocked blood vessel due to ischemia and hypoxia is still reversible before the nerve neurones become entirely necrotic. Scalp acupuncture applied then at the motor area may dilate the blood vessels around the lesion, enhance the establishment of collateral blood circulation, improve the supply of nutrients to the nerve cells and promote the recovery of the function of damaged brain tissue.

(b) Location of Thrombosis and Therapeutic Effect

In 1971, the author and his colleagues found that there was also a close relationship between the therapeutic effect of scalp acupuncture and the location of thrombosis, that is, scalp acupuncture will achieve a better therapeutic effect in patients with cerebral thrombosis at the cortical branches of the cerebral artery than in those with cerebral thrombosis at the deep branches or the trunk of the big arteries. This conclusion has been repeatedly verified by clinical practice.

The Dalian Railway Hospital in northeast China's Liaoning Province treated 91 patients of cerebral thrombosis with scalp acupuncture. Of the 68 patients with thrombosis at the cortical branches of the middle cerebral artery, 45 were completely cured, accounting for 66.17 percent; 15 witnessed apparent improvement in their symptoms, accounting for 22.1 percent; one witnessed a lesser degree of agreement and another one did not see any improvement. But of 23 patients with thrombosis at the deep branches of the middle cerebral artery, only seven were cured, accounting for 30.43 percent; another seven witnessed apparent improvement in their symptoms, accounting for 30.43 percent; eight witnessed a lesser degree of improvement, accounting for 34.78 percent; and one did not see any improvement. This indicates that a better therapeutic result can be achieved in patients with the thrombosis lying at the cortical branches.

To further prove that a better therapeutic result in cases in which the lesions are closer to the surface skin of the scalp, the author and his colleagues selected 20 acute cases of cerebral thrombosis characterized by monoplegia. Moreover, CT scan was used to identify the lesions at the cortical branches. Scalp acupuncture was applied 2-12 hours after the onset of the disease at the motor area on the same side as the lesions by prompt inserting and twisting the needles. As a result, nine cases were cured, accounting for 45 percent; marked improvement were achieved in 10 cases, accounting for 50 percent; and a lesser degree of improvement was witnessed in one case, accounting for 5 percent. The reason for the better therapeutic effect is that the lesions in the cerebral cortex locate closer to the surface of the scalp, the needling stimulation at the motor area on the scalp can produce a more direct action to the blood vessels of the underlying brain cortex to improve their elasticity, dilate their lumen, increase the volume of blood flow, improve the blood circulation of brain, raise the partial pressure of oxygen in the cerebral tissue, increase the supply of nutrients to the nerve cells around the lesion and promote the repairing of the brain tissue.

(c) Severity of Limp Paralysis and Therapeutic Effect

In 1971, the author and his colleagues found that there was also a close relationship between the severity of paralysis of the limbs and the therapeutic effect, that is, scalp acupuncture would produce better therapeutic effect in patients with partial paralysis of the limbs than in patients with complete paralysis of the limps. This hypothesis has been proved by the extensive clinical practice. For instance, the Tangshan Steel Company Hospital has achieved a satisfactory result in treating cases of a mild cerebral thrombosis with scalp acupuncture.

To study the relationship between the severity of paralysis caused by cerebral thrombosis and the cure rate of scalp acupuncture, the Hospital of Traditional Chinese Medicine affiliated to the Shandong Medical College observed 65 cases of paralysis of upper limbs and 67 cases of paralysis of lower limbs, both caused by cerebral thrombosis.

Of the group of patients with paralysis of the upper limbs, 10 out of the 17 cases with mild paralysis, or 58.8 percent, were cured; two out of the of the 25 cases with medium paralysis, or 8 percent, were cured; and none out of the 23 patients with severe paralysis were cured.

Of the group of patients with paralysis of the lower limbs, 14 out of the 33 cases with mild paralysis, or 42.4 percent, were cured; none out of the 14 cases with medium paralysis was cured; and three out of the 20 cases with severe paralysis, or 15.4 percent, were cured.

The above statistics show that scalp acupuncture obtains a higher cure rate in mild cases of paralysis caused by cerebral thrombosis.

(d) Time of Appearance of Therapeutic Effect

It has been proved that scalp acupuncture is an effective therapy for cerebral thrombosis. It can produce an immediate therapeutic result in some cases. For example, the Hainan People's Hospital once used scalp acupuncture to treat 20 patients with cerebral thrombosis, of whom 10, or 50 percent, were cured; eight, or 40 percent, were greatly relieved; and two, or 10 percent, were improved. Of the 20 patients, apparent improvement was witnessed in 11 immediately after the first round of treatment by scalp acupuncture.

Case Report:

(1) Yin, female, 50 years old, from Jishan County, Shanxi Province.

Chief complaint: Hemiplegia on the right side for 40 days.

Case history: Having got up in early morning on November 30, 1970, the patient felt that the movement of her right limbs was impaired—her right hand could not hold things and her right leg could not stand straight and walk.

Physical examination: The patient had a clear state of mind and could express herself. The right arm could move a little but with difficulty to hold up and extend the right the hand. The right leg could raise up slight but with difficulty to bend, stretch, stand erect and walk. The deep reflexes were exaggerated and the pathological neurological signs were negative. A systolic murmur of third grade was diagnosed over the tricuspid valves. The Kline test was positive (+++).

Diagnosis: Syphilitic endarteritis of cerebral artery with thrombosis.

Selected stimulating area: Upper three-fifths of the left motor area.

Treatment: After the needles were inserted and twisted for the first round, the patient witnessed a hot feeling running like a stream reaching out to the fingers and toes. After twisting of the needle went on for three minutes, the hot feeling was enhanced and the patient had a more comfortable feeling in her affected limbs. Then, the needles were removed. The patient found her right arm could raise up normally and she could walk at a normal gait without any other's support.

(2) Wang, male, 63 years old, from Yuncheng, Shanxi Province.

Chief complaint: Hemiplegia on the right side for three days.

Case history: Awaking from noon nap three days before, the patient felt numbness in his right hand. Moreover, the symptom developed quickly and soon the movement of his arm was impaired—he could not write and play the abacus.

Medical examination: The patient had a clear state of mind, his speech was slightly garbled, and his tongue slightly deviated to the right side. The right arm could raise up to the level of the shoulder, the right hand could extend to 100 degrees, the fingers could bent back to a point 2 centimetres from the palm, and the thumb and index finger could not pinch. The right hand could not hold a pen. While writing, he could only pinch the pen with the thumb, index and middle fingers and slide the pen over the paper by moving the elbow instead of moving the wrist, and as a result, the characters he wrote were messed up as shown in Fig. 3-1. The gripping strength of the right hand was 9 kg while that of the left hand 30 kg. The tendon reflex was exaggerated and the Hoffmann's sign was positive. As the patient felt weak in the right leg, he had an apparent hemiplegic gait. The blood pressure was normal.

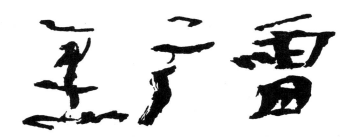

Fig. 3-1   Characters written before treatment

Diagnosis: Cerebral arteriosclerosis with cerebral thrombosis of left middle cerebral artery, partial paralysis of right limbs and partial aphasia.

Selected stimulating area: Motor area and motor and sensory area of foot on the left side.

Treatment: Scalp acupuncture was applied once a day. After the first round of treatment, the progression of the disease was brought under control and the physical signs were immediately improved—the right hand could stretch and bend normally, with its gripping strength increasing to 16 kg; the thumb and index finger of the right hand could pinch together and the right arm could raise to 160 degrees; and the speech became normal. After the fifth round of treatment, the right arm could raise up normally and the gripping strength of the right hand increased to 20 kg. The right hand could stretch and bend nimbly and the pinching force between the thumb and index finger was strong enough to hold a pen to write better characters as shown in Fig. 3-2. After the sixth round of treatment, the patient could speak clearly; the muscular strength of the right upper and lower limbs recovered to normal and the gripping strength of the right hand increased

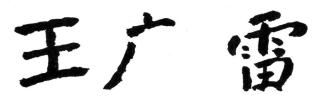

Fig. 3-2   Characters written after the fifth round of treatment

to 30 kg.

(3) Liu, female, 57 years old, from Yuncheng, Shanxi Province.

Chief complaint: Hemiplegia of right side for one and a half years.

Case history: In the morning of February 2, 1977, the patient suddenly developed paralysis in her right limbs together with temporary unconsciousness. The right arm could not move and she could not walk because of weakness of the right leg. Treatment by both traditional Chinese medicine and Western medicine had helped relieve the symptoms to a certain degree, but had not produced a complete cure.

Physical examination: The patient had a clear state of mind. Yet, her speech was slightly garbled. The right nasolabial groove was shallower than normal and the tongue deviated slightly to the right when protruding. The right arm was weak and the gripping strength of the right hand was 8 kg (20 kg for left hand). The right hand could stretch to 160 degrees, but the fingers could not separate from one another. The thumb and index finger of the right hand could not pinch together to hold a pen. She could walk a little with the support of a walking stick, showing an apparent hemiplegic gait.

Diagnosis: Cerebral thrombosis with partial hemiplegia of the right limbs.

Selected stimulating areas: Left motor area and motor and sensory area of foot.

Treatment: Scalp acupuncture was applied once a day. After the first round of treatment, the patient could stretch the fingers of her right hand. After the second round of treatment, the fingers could be separated from one another and her right leg became strong enough that she could walk 100 meters without any support. After the sixth round of treatment, the patient could stand up by herself from a low stool. And after the eighth round of treatment, she could nimbly flex and stretch her right hand and separate the fingers. The gripping strength of her right hand increased to 13 kg, and she could hold a pen firmly to write better characters.

(4) A Saudi Arabian man.

Chief complaint: Left hemiplegia for one and half a year.

Case history: In October 1991, the patient suddenly developed hemiplegia in his left limbs without loss of consciousness.

Physical examination: The patient was mentally clear and could speak normally. The left nasolabial groove was shallower than normal and the tongue deviated to the left side when protruded. The left arm could raise up to the level of the shoulder and the left hand always took a semi-flexed posture because the fingers could not flex and stretch. The muscular tonus was increased and the Hoffmann's sign for the left hand was positive. The movement of left lower limb was impaired and the movement below the ankle joint was limited. The patient walked at an apparent hemiplegic gait.

Diagnosis: Partial hemiplegia of the left side caused by cerebral thrombosis.

Selected stimulating areas: Right motor area and motor and sensory area of foot.

Treatment: Scalp acupuncture was applied once a day and some therapeutic effect was achieved after several rounds of treatment. After the 22nd round of treatment, the patient was able to raise his left arm to a normal height, the fingers of the left hand could be nimbly flexed and stretched, and the left leg was powerful enough to walk at a stable gait.

(2) Cerebral Haemorrhage

Cerebral haemorrhage refers to bleeding in the parenchyma of the brain due to rupture of the cerebral blood vessels. In traditional Chinese medicine, it is also called haemorrhagic apoplexy due to attack of wind at the internal organs. It is also a very common cerebrovascular disease with an incidence second only to cerebral thrombosis. A higher morbidity of this disease is witnessed among people around 50 years of age with high blood pressure.

Usually, the disease is caused by a sudden rise of blood pressure after emotional disturbance, extreme excitement, nervousness, difficult defecation or heavy physical exertion in patients with hypertension and atherosclerosis.

The disease can be divided into two types: Haemorrhage of internal capsule (basal ganglia) and haemorrhage of cortical branches of the cerebral artery.

Haemorrhage of internal capsule: The onset of disease is prompt and the patients may have long coma, hemiplegia, hemidysesthenia and hemi-anopsia.

Haemorrhage of cortical branches: The onset of disease is quick and most patients may have a short-term coma. The severity of paralysis thus caused may be varied due to bleeding at different parts of the cortex. For example, bleeding in a cortical branch of the middle cerebral artery may cause monoplegia of the upper limb or more serious symptoms in the upper limb, and some patients may also show the symptoms due to stimulation of the cerebral cortex, such as epilepsy.

Selected stimulating areas: The motor area, sensory area and the motor and sensory area of foot on the opposite side of the physical signs.

Treatment: At the acute stage with coma, routine emergent treatment should be given. After consciousness is restored and the patients' conditions become stable, scalp acupuncture is then applied.

It has been proved that scalp acupuncture can produce a marked therapeutic effect to cerebral haemorrhage. It can effect a complete cure for 20 percent of the patients, and for another 30 percent it can bring a marked improvement in their physical symptoms.

The therapeutic result of scalp acupuncture is closely related to the location of the bleeding. Usually, it is poor in patients with bleeding in the internal capsule, although in a few patients it may produce an apparent improvement. In some patients, the therapeutic effect cannot be seen before a long period of treatment.

In patients with bleeding in the cortical branches of the cerebral artery, scalp acupuncture can produce a satisfactory and quicker therapeutic result. Some patients may be cured and can walk without any support after only one or several rounds of treatment.

The mechanism of scalp acupuncture for relieving hemiplegia, numbness and aphasia caused by cerebral haemorrhage is many sided, and the important one is to promote the absorption of blood escaped from the blood vessels and the relief of physical symptoms.

Of a total of 1,659 cases of cerebral haemorrhage treated with scalp acupuncture, 397 were basically cured, accounting for 23.93 percent; 576 were apparently improved, accounting for 34.72 percent; 579 showed different degrees of improvement, accounting for 34.9 percent; 105 did not show any effect, accounting for 6.33 percent; one deteriorated; and one died.

The following is a general discussion about important factors affecting the therapeutic result of scalp acupuncture for cerebral haemorrhage.

(a) Clinical course: Clinical experience proves that applying scalp acupuncture treatment at an earlier date after the patients' conditions become stable can produce a better therapeutic result.

(b) Location of bleeding: In 1971, the author and his colleagues already found scalp acupuncture produced a poor therapeutic effect in patients with bleeding in the internal capsule and a better therapeutic result in patients with bleeding in the cortical branches of the cerebral artery. For some patients with bleeding in the cortical branches, one or several rounds of treatment could enable them to stand up and walk. For instance, in 1971 the Dalian Railway Hospital used scalp acupuncture to treat eight patients with bleeding in the cortical branches and 66 patients with bleeding in the internal capsule. The eight patients with bleeding in the cortical branches were all cured, while of the 66 patients with bleeding in the internal capsule, 14 were cured, accounting for 21.2 percent; 16 were remarkably improved, accounting for 24.2 percent; 32 were improved by lesser degrees, accounting for 48.5 percent; and four did not show any improvement, accounting for 6.1 percent.

(c) Time needed for therapeutic effect to manifest itself: Scalp acupuncture can produce a very quick curative effect for patients of cerebral haemorrhage. In June, 1971, the author used scalp acupuncture to treat a patient of cerebral haemorrhage. By then, the patient had suffered from the disease for 24 hours, and his right arm was completed paralysed and could not raise up 10 centimetres. Yet, he had a clear state of mind. The diagnosis of cerebral haemorrhage was proven by the blood colour in the cerebrospinal fluid (CSF). Just after one round scalp acupuncture treatment at the left motor area and the motor and sensory area of foot, the patient could immediately stand up and walk. In Taiwan, Chen Kang and Liu Xitai treated 23 patients of cerebral haemorrhage with scalp acupuncture and all patients were completely recovered. Among the patients was a 65-year-old foreign woman with the family name of Hans. She had suffered from right hemiplegia, numbness and loss of pain as well as tactile sensation for two months. Immediately after the first round of treatment at the left motor area and sensory area, she was able to flex and extend her right arm and leg, stand up and walk a little. She completely recovered after the fourth round of treatment. Based on their clinical experience, Chen and Liu wrote a paper titled Experience to Treat Cerebral Haemorrhage with Scalp Acupuncture and published it in an acupuncture journal in the United States.

Case Report:
(1) Apraxia after cerebral haemorrhage
Xu, male, 41 years old, from Huaxian County, Guangdong Province.
One day in 1962, the patient suddenly contracted coma accompanied with

paralysis of the right limbs. Treatment by local physicians relieved to some extent the symptoms, except for weakness of the right arm and apraxia of the right hand. The physical examination proved weakness of the right limbs, although the patient could walk. The right arm could move within normal range. But the gripping strength of the right hand was slightly poor—it could not unbutton clothes and hold a pen. After just one round of treatment with scalp acupuncture, the patient could immediately unbutton the clothes, hold a pen to write and even pick up a coin from the floor.

(2) Cerebral haemorrhage

Wang, male, 54 years old, from Jishan County, Shanxi Province.

The patient suddenly fell into a coma while doing some sort of physical labour and was brought to the hospital. He recovered from the blackout 24 hours after the onset of the disease. Physical examination then showed he had a clear state of mind, motor aphasia and complete paralysis of right arm. The right leg could be lifted 10 cm high and the CSF had a red colour.

After the first round of treatment by scalp acupuncture at left motor area, the patient could freely raise, flex and stretch the right leg, and could stand for 20 seconds. After the second round of treatment, the muscular strength of right leg was further increased and the patient could walk over four meters without any support. After 29 rounds of treatment, the patient could move his right arm within normal range and walk normally. In addition, speech was basically restored. Follow-up visits for two months showed that patient could do common physical jobs.

(3) Right hemiplegia accompanied by high intracranial pressure after cerebral haemorrhage

Li, female, 34 years old, from Wanrong County, Shanxi Province.

Chief complaint: Right hemiplegia for 19 days.

Case history: The patient had suffered from headache and nausea for some time. On April 1, 1979, her mind suddenly become muddled and she fell into complete coma 20 minutes later. More than an hour later, the patient recovered consciousness, but contracted complete hemiplegia in the right limbs. She was brought to a hospital in Yuncheng five days later. Lumbar puncture in the hospital showed an increase of intracranial pressure to 320 mm of water and the CSF had a yellowish colour with a RBC count of 785/cubic mm. Successive IV infusion of low molecular dextran solution failed to relieve her sufferings.

Physical examination: The patient had a clear state of mind and could speak normally. The function of the cranial nerves was normal. The right hand could flex and stretch normally, but the gripping strength of the right hand was only 4 kg (34 kg for the left hand). The Hoffmann's sign was negative. The right arm could be raised to the level of the xiphoid process and the right leg was completely paralysed. The muscular tonus increased, the knee jerk exaggerated, and the Barbinski's sign was negative. The temperature, pain and cutaneous sensations of the right half of the body were all normal. The heart beat was regular and 70 per minute, and the blood pressure was 100/70 mmHg. There was no valvular murmur in heart and rales in lungs.

Funduscopic examination showed congestion of bilateral optic discs with blurred margins and radiating in appearance, with the abnormality being more obvious in the left eye. The left optic disc was more bulged, by 3-4 D than the right one. The arterioles of fundus were normal, but the venules of fundus were dilated and distorted, A:V=1:2. There was no arteriovenous crossing sign and no haemorrhage and exudate. The light reflex of central fovea of macula was clearly visible.

The arteriogram of left carotid artery showed that the internal carotid artery and the anterior and middle cerebral arteries were normal.

The electromyograms of bilateral superficial flexor muscles of fingers, deltoid muscles, medial femoral vastus muscles and anterior tibial muscles were recorded by a Denmark-made electromyograph of 4 channels with a time base of 20 ms and an electric potential of 500 μv through a concentric pin-shaped electrode.

1) Motor points of bilateral superficial flexor muscles of fingers: The peak value of left hand was 3,000 μv and that of the right hand reached 2,500 μv when both hands were flexed (Fig. 3-3).

2) Motor points of bilateral deltoid muscles: The peak value of the left arm reached 3,200 μv and that of the right arm 150 μv when both arms were stretched (Fig. 3-4).

3) Motor points of bilateral medial femoral vastus muscles: The peak value of the left leg reached 3,200 μv and there was no electric discharge for the right leg (Fig. 3-5).

4) Motor points of bilateral anterior tibial muscles: The peak value of the left leg reached 2,700 μv and there was no electric discharge for the right leg (Fig. 3-6).

Selected stimulating areas: Upper three-fifths of left motor area and left motor and sensory area of foot.

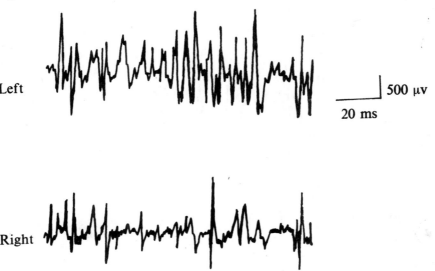

Left

500 μv

20 ms

Right

Fig. 3-3   Electromyogram of fingers of both hands

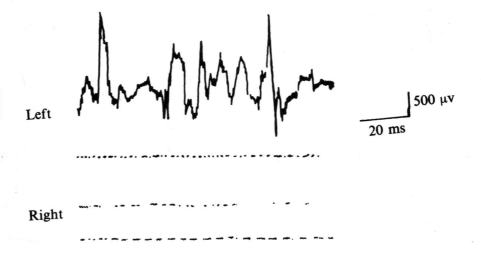

Fig. 3-4   Electromyogram of bilateral deltoid muscles

Treatment: The treatment was applied once a day. After six rounds of treatment, the clinical symptoms were greatly relieved—the right arm could raise to a normal height, the gripping strength of the right hand increased to 26 kg, the right leg could move normally and the patient could walk four or five steps without any support. After 15 rounds of treatment, the muscle strength of the right arm returned to normal, the gripping strength of the right hand increased to 32 kg, the

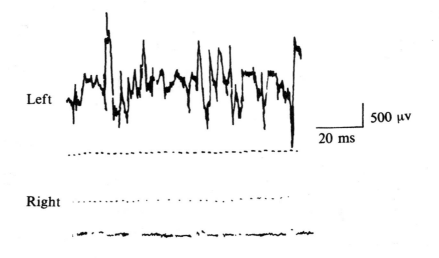

Fig. 3-5   Electromyogram of bilateral medial femoral vastus muscles

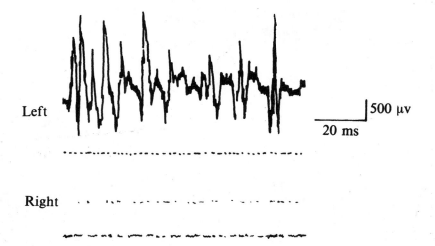

Fig. 3-6   Electromyogram of bilateral anterior tibial muscles

movement of the various joints of the right leg became more nimble. But the movement of the right ankle joint was still limited and the muscle strength of right toes was still poor.

Re-examination by electromyography showed that the peak value had increased to 3,200 μv, 2,800 μv and 2,600 μv for the right superficial flexor muscle of fingers, medial femoral vastus muscle and anterior tibial muscle respectively (Figs. 3-7, 3-8, 3-9 and 3-10).

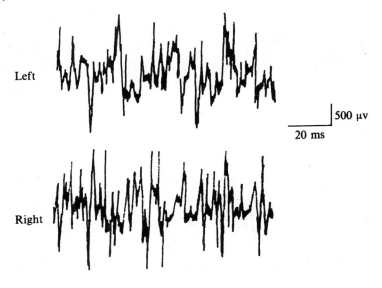

Fig. 3-7   Electromyogram of both hands after treatment

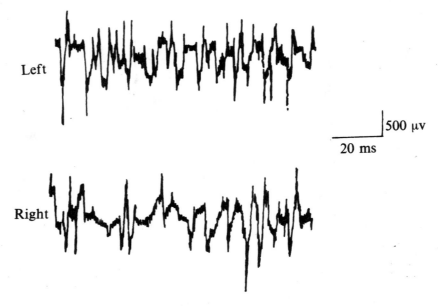

Fig. 3-8   Electromyogram bilateral deltoid muscles after treatment

The optic disc of the left eye was 2 D higher than that of the right eye and the border of left optic disc remained still blurred. But the margins of the right optic disc restored its clearness. The intracranial pressure reduced to 230 mmH$_2$O. The CSF was clear and transparent, the content of protein was 10 mg% and no RBC was found in the CSF under microscope.

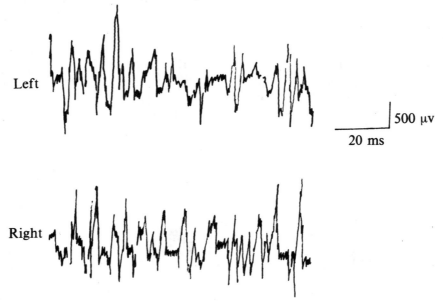

Fig. 3-9   Electromyogram bilateral medial femoral
vastus muscles after treatment

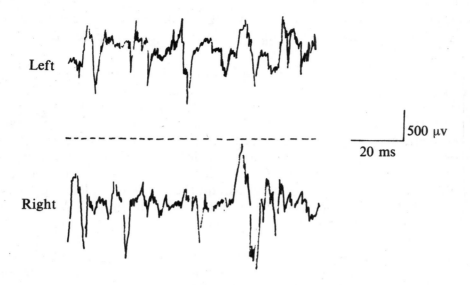

Left

500 μv

20 ms

Right

Fig. 3-10   Electromyogram bilateral anterior tibial muscles after treatment

(3) Cerebral Embolism

Cerebral embolism is a cerebrovascular disease due to the blockade of the carotid artery or cerebral artery by foreign body (solid, liquid or gas) and it is more common in patients with stenosis of mitral valves of the heart and in patients at middle age. The onset of the disease is prompt without any prodromal symptoms and the disease may turn into a crisis within a very short time or even a few seconds. In some patients it may deteriorate progressively within several days. The incidence of the disease is about 0.04 percent. As it usually occurs in the anterior portion of basilar arterial ring, it is often manifested as facial paralysis, monoplegia of the upper limbs, hemiplegia, aphasia and focal convulsion, which are usual clinical symptoms of lesions in the internal carotid artery.

Selected stimulating areas: The motor area, sensory area and the motor and sensory area of foot on the opposite side of the physical signs.

Treatment: In patients with cardiac dysfunction, scalp acupuncture should be applied until the clinical symptoms are brought under control.

Scalp acupuncture is slightly less effective for patients of cerebral embolism than it is for patients of cerebral thrombosis. About one-third of patients of cerebral embolism can be cured and marked improvement can be achieved in another one-third. In most patients, the improvement is observed after 5-8 rounds of treatment, but in a few patients a satisfactory result can be obtained after just one round of treatment. The cure rate is higher in patients with a short clinical course. There is a close relationship between therapeutic result and the location of the embolus.

Of the 304 cases of cerebral embolism treated with scalp acupuncture, 90 were cured, accounting for 29.6 percent; marked improvement was achieved in 85, accounting for 27.96 percent; lesser degrees of improvement were observed in 94, accounting for 30.92 percent; 33 did not see any effect, accounting for 10.85 percent; and two of the patients died, accounting for 0.65 percent.

Case Report:

Qu, male, 46 years old, from Jishan County, Shanxi Province.

Chief complaint: Right hemiplegia for two days.

Case history: Two days before, the patient suddenly developed numbness in his right hand, followed by quick development of hemiplegia of the right limbs without coma and disturbance of speech, urination and defecation.

Physical examination: The patient had a clear state of mind and normal speech. The right nasolabial groove was shallower than normal and the tongue deviated to the right when protruding. The right arm and leg were completely paralysed. The patient had a history of rheumatic heart disease with mitral stenosis and undergone an operation on the heart.

Diagnosis: Cerebral embolism.

Selected stimulating area: Left motor area.

Treatment: Scalp acupuncture was applied once a day. After 60 rounds of treatment, the paralysis of right limbs had completely gone and the patient could take care of himself. The gripping strength of the right hand increased to 30 kg.

(4) Bulbar Paralysis

If the medulla oblongata is affected in injury of the brain, disturbance of speech and dysphagia may develop. This is called bulbar paralysis, as the medulla oblongata is round like a ball.

According to location of the lesion and clinical manifestations, bulbar paralysis can be divided into two types.

(a) True bulbar paralysis: The lesion usually locates on one side of the medulla oblongata and it is often caused by cerebral thrombosis or insufficiency of blood supply from the vertebrobasilar artery. It may have such manifestations as dyslalia, dysphagia and disappearance of pharyngeal reflex. But, the disturbance of the functions of cerebral cortex is not obvious.

(b) False bulbar paralysis: The lesions locate on both sides of the corticomedullary tract and they are usually caused by thrombosis in the vascular system of the internal carotid artery. Usually, the patients have two attacks of cerebral thrombosis and the manifestations include disturbance of speech, dysphagia, choking when eating, dripping of saliva and limited movement of the soft palate. The pharyngeal reflex exists while the palmomental reflex and sucking reflex are positive. The functions of cerebral cortex are seriously impaired and the patients may cry now and laugh then.

Scalp Acupuncture Treatment: For true bulbar paralysis, the balance areas on both sides are selected as the main stimulating areas and the madness controlling area as the supplementary area to treat the thrombosis in the medulla oblongata.

For false bulbar paralysis, the lower two-fifths of the motor areas and the balance areas on both sides are chosen to treat the thrombosis in the cerebral cortex, the subcortical region and the corticomedullary tract.

Of the 51 cases of bulbar paralysis treated with scalp acupuncture, 31 were cured, accounting for 60.78 percent; 16 were markedly relieved, accounting for 31.37 percent; and four were improved at lesser degrees, accounting for 7.84 percent.

As the above discussion shows, scalp acupuncture is indeed effective in treating cerebrovascular diseases, such as cerebral thrombosis and cerebral haemorrhage.

Chinese medical workers have also used scalp acupuncture to treat 11,126 patients with clinical symptoms of cerebrovascular diseases but not definitely diagnosed. Among them, 4,128 were cured, accounting for 37.1 percent of the total; 3,862 were markedly relieved, accounting for 34.71 percent; 2,604 were relieved by lesser degrees, accounting for 23.4 percent; and 522 did not show any improvement, accounting for 4.78 percent.

Therefore, scalp acupuncture can produce a satisfactory therapeutic result when used to treat patients with clinical symptoms of cerebrovascular diseases, despite the lack of a definite diagnosis.

II. Cerebral Injury

Cerebral injury refers to common external trauma. Although cerebral injuries make up 20 percent of total physical injuries, they rank the first place in mortality.

In clinical practice, cerebral injuries are divided into the open and closed types. The open type refers to injuries in which the pia mater and brain tissue are exposed after the scalp, skull and dura mater are lacerated and broken, while the closed type refers to injuries in which at least one of the three protective structures—the scalp, skull and dura mater—remains intact and offers protection to the pia mater and brain tissue from being directly exposed to the external environment.

Organic injury of the brain caused by external violence is called contusion and laceration of the brain. At the time when an injury is inflicted, the patient may have coma and develop such localized physical signs as hemiplegia, numbness and aphasia.

Selected stimulating areas: The motor area, sensory area and the motor and sensory area of foot on the opposite side of the physical symptoms.

Treatment: At the acute stage of the injury, emergent surgical measures should first be adopted to bring the patient's conditions under control. After the patient's consciousness is restored, scalp acupuncture can then be applied to treat the physical symptoms of hemiplegia, numbness and aphasia. According to the theory of Western medicine, the brain neurones cannot regenerate once seriously damaged. Yet, scalp acupuncture, when applied at the motor area and sensory area, can produce a quick and effective cure to hemiplegia, numbness and aphasia caused by contusion and laceration of brain. Moreover, it has been proved particularly effective for closed-type cerebral injuries of infants.

Of the 540 cases of cerebral injury treated with scalp acupuncture, 199 were basically cured, accounting for 36.85 percent; 129 were markedly relieved, accounting for 23.88 percent; 177 were improved by varying degrees, accounting for 32.77 percent; and 35 did not see any effect, accounting for 6.4 percent.

To further study the effect of scalp acupuncture in treating infant hemiplegia caused by contusion and laceration of the brain, from 1983 to 1985 the author and his colleagues selected seven boys—all suffering from injuries of the brain—and made a systematic observation. The boys ranged from six months to six years old and had a clinical course of 2-4 days. In all cases, scalp acupuncture was applied once a day at the upper three-fifths of the motor area and the motor and sensory area of foot on the opposite side of the lesions.

Course of treatment: On average, 16.5 rounds of treatment were given to each of the seven little patients (116 rounds in total).

Therapeutic effect: After the first round of treatment, therapeutic effect was observed in six of the patients, accounting for 84.2 percent. In the end, six cases were cured, accounting for 84.2 percent; and remaining one was greatly relieved.

Case Report:

(1) Pei, a boy of 10 months old, from Hejin County, Shanxi Province.

Chief complaint: Left hemiplegia due to contusion of the brain for three days.

Case history: On June 29, 1983, the boy accidentally fell down from the arms of his parents, with his head hitting the ground. As a result, he developed paraplegia of the left limbs when recovered from coma.

Physical examination: Complete paralysis of left limbs.

Treatment: Scalp acupuncture was applied once a day at the right motor area and the motor and sensory area of foot. After the second round of treatment, the boy could move his left limbs. After the eighth round of treatment, the paralysis completely disappeared. Follow-up checks in the ensuing two years showed the baby grew up normally.

In 1985, the boy was again subject to a contusion and laceration of the brain with right hemiplegia. He was again cured by scalp acupuncture.

A follow-up visit made in October 1990 proved that the child was very healthy and all his limbs moved nimbly.

(2) Fan, a boy of six years old.

Chief complaint: Right hemiplegia due to cerebral injury for three days.

Case history: On November 3, 1985, the boy fell on ground with his head being badly injured. He immediately blacked out. After regaining consciousness, he developed right hemiplegia.

Physical examination: The patient had a clear state of mind and could speak fluently. The right nasolabial groove was shallower than normal. The right limbs were completely paralysed, with muscular strength being "0" grade. The Barbinski's and Hoffmann's signs of the right limbs were positive.

Treatment: Scalp acupuncture was applied once a day at the upper three-fifths of the motor area and the motor and sensory area of foot on the left side. After the first round of treatment, the child could move his right limbs slightly. After the 12th round of treatment, paralysis of the right limbs completely disappeared and the child could nimbly perform such delicate jobs as picking up a needle.

A follow-up visit in October 1990 showed that the child was perfectly healthy.

III. Intracranial Infection

Here, intracranial infection refers to inflammation of the brain and meninges due to various causes and the different kinds of encephalitis.

The onset of encephalitis and meningitis is prompt in most cases and usually accompanied by high fever, coma or convulsion. The inflammatory change of CSF can prove the diagnosis of intracranial infection. For most patients, the clinical manifestations can be controlled and improved by routine medical therapies. But for some patients the sequelae due to damage of the parenchymal tissues of the brain, such as the paralysis of limbs, numbness, aphasia and impaired vision, may remain for a long time.

Selected stimulating areas: The motor area, the sensory area and the motor and sensory area of foot on the opposite side of the physical symptoms.

Treatment: At the acute stage when there is high fever and coma, the patients should first be treated with routine medical methods, and scalp acupuncture can only applied to treat the remaining paralysis of limbs, numbness, aphasia and blindness after the patients regain consciousness. The therapeutic results vary greatly. For some patients, their trouble can be cured by scalp acupuncture. But for some others, the therapeutic result cannot be observed in a short period of time.

Of the 1,255 cases of nine different kinds of intracranial infection treated with scalp acupuncture, 314 were cured, accounting for 25.01 percent. In 1,106 cases, scalp acupuncture has been proved to be effective. Of the 1,255 patients, there were 902 cases of encephalitis, of which 171 were cured, accounting for 18.95 percent; there were 141 cases of encephalitis B, of which 66 were cured, accounting for 46.8 percent; and there were 58 cases of toxic encephalitis, of which 31 were cured, accounting for 53.11 percent. The cure rate of encephalitis B and toxic encephalitis was respectively 3.46-fold and 3.82-fold higher than that of encephalitis.

Case Report:
(1) Recovery stage of encephalitis

Pan, a girl of two years old, from Wanrong County, Shanxi Province.

Chief complaint: High fever and coma for half a month.

Case history: In late March 1971, the girl suddenly got a temperature of 40 degrees centigrade accompanied by coma and convulsion. After medical treatment for half a month, she regained consciousness but became blind. At the same time, she developed complete motor aphasia and paralysis of four limbs.

Physical examination: The patient had a clear state of mind but dilatation of both pupils, complete motor aphasia, paralysis of the limbs and weakness of the neck.

Selected stimulating area: Motor and optic areas on both sides.

Treatment: Scalp acupuncture was applied once a day. After five rounds of treatment, the girl could see things and the paralysed limbs could move. After 20 rounds of treatment, the movement of the limbs became normal and she could stand up by her own. Her health was gradually restored.

Follow-up visits were made from July 1972 through March 1991. The girl's physical and mental development had been normal, so been her mentality and facial expression; her speech was fluent and her sight was good.

(2) Right hemiplegia after tuberculous meningitis

Zhang, a boy of four years old, from Yuncheng, Shanxi Province.

Chief complaint: Right hemiplegia for over three years.

Case history: In January, 1978, the boy got a high temperature of 40 degrees centigrade and vomited, but did not lose consciousness. A diagnosis of tuberculous meningitis was verified by lumbar puncture. Ensuing treatment relieved to a certain degree the conditions. Yet, 10 days later, the boy developed repeated involuntary convulsions in the right limbs in short intervals, once every few minutes. Shortly after, the movement of the right limbs was impaired and paralysed. Although medical treatment helped bring the muscular convulsions under control, the right limbs remained paralysed.

Physical examination: The boy had a clear state of mind and could speak normally. The right arm was completely paralysed with an increase of muscular tonus, and the right leg was too weak to stand up and walk, even with the support of another person. The toes remained always flexed and could not stretched.

Selected stimulating areas: Upper three-fifths of the motor area and the motor and sensory area of foot on the left side of the body.

Treatment: Scalp acupuncture was applied once a day. After the first round of treatment, the patient was able to walk with the support of another person, as he could move his right leg. After the third round of treatment, he could flex and stretch his right hand to pick up something. After the fourth round of treatment, the boy could walk independently and raise his right hand to touch the head.

(3) Toxic encephalitis

Yang, a girl of four years old, from Yuncheng, Shanxi Province.

Chief complaint: Paralysis of all limbs for 26 days after an attack of toxic bacillary dysentery.

Case history: On September 1, 1978, the girl defecated blood and pus, but had no coma and fever, with the body temperature at 36.8 degrees centigrade. Three days later, she lost the ability to speak and move her limbs. Although the bloody and pussy diarrhoea stopped 13 days later, still she could not speak, raise her head and sit up because of weakness in the neck and waist.

Physical examination: The patient showed a pale complexion. She could not raise her head, sit up, move her limbs and answer questions of the physician. The fingers of both hands were always flexed.

Selected stimulating areas: Motor area, and motor and sensory area of foot on both sides.

Treatment: Scalp acupuncture was applied once a day or every two or three days. After 10 rounds of treatment, an obvious improvement of the weakness of the neck was observed; she was able to raise her head and could move her limbs within normal range. After 15 rounds of treatment, she could say her name and call "Mom" and "Dad." After 52 rounds of treatment, her ability to speak returned to normal, so did the muscular strength of the found limbs. The movement of her fingers was nimble and she could walk independently.

IV. Lesions in Basal Ganglia

1. Chorea

The choreic diseases contain the chorea minor, progressive chronic chorea, hemichorea, senile chorea and chorea gravidarum. Among them the chorea minor is more common.

(1) Chorea Minor

Chorea minor, also called chorea rheumatism, chorea infectiosa or Sydenham's chorea, is a clinical manifestation of acute rheumatism more common in children.

In most cases, chorea minor is a subacute disease with choreic movement typical of diseases in the basal ganglia. At the early stage, the symptoms are not very obvious. The children tend to be just more irritable and less quiet. By and by, it will be increasingly difficult for them to concentrate in their studies; the movement of their limbs will become increasingly clumsy; their gait will become more and more unsteady; they will find it more and more difficult to hold things firmly and their handwriting will be badly scrawled. Parents and teachers might mistakenly consider them as being nervous or naughty children. As the disease progresses, an involuntary quick, jerky, irregular and nonsensical movement may first appear in one limb and spread to another limb of the same side and finally to the limbs of the contralateral side. If the facial muscles are also affected, the patients may frequently knit their eyebrows and wink their eyes. Light hemiplegia and derangement may occur in some patients.

Selected stimulating areas: Chorea and tremor controlling area on the opposite side of the symptoms, or on both sides if the symptoms appear on both sides of the body.

Treatment: Scalp acupuncture is applied once a day. Usually, therapeutic effect can be observed after six or seven rounds of treatment, and occasionally after just one round. The therapeutic effect is more satisfactory for juvenile chorea than for other types of chorea. The increase of red blood cell (RBC) sediment rate may return to normal level along with the relief of the symptoms.

Case Report:

(1) Chorea minor

Wen, a girl of 15 years old, from Jishan County, Shanxi Province.

Chief complaint: Irregular involuntary movement of all limbs for 40 days.

Case history: On February 22, 1971, the girl was found to repeatedly stretch and abduct both her hands involuntarily while working in the field. She accidentally cut the crop seedings while doing hoeing job. As the disease turned more serious, she began to knit her eyebrows and wink her eyes, and her limbs always moved involuntarily. She found it difficult to sleep, sit erect and walk around. Eventually, she lost the ability to take care of herself.

Physical examination: The patient could not sit still. When lying in bed, she constantly tossed over with the waist and hip moving to and fro. So, she might fall from bed if not looked after by another person. She also constantly knitted her eyebrows, winked her eyes and moved her limbs unintentionally.

Selected stimulating areas: Chorea and tremor controlling areas on both sides.

Treatment: Scalp acupuncture was applied once a day. After 16 rounds of treatment, her facial expression returned to normal and the involuntary movement of limbs stopped. After 24 rounds of treatment, she regained the ability to take care of herself. She was discharged from the hospital on May 20, 1971.

Follow-up visits by the author in 1972-92 showed that the girl was all right mentally and physically. She could even do some farm work.

(2) Chorea minor with increased RBC sediment rate

Li, a young female of 21 years old, from Wanrong County, Shanxi Province. Chief complaint: Involuntary movement of the limbs for 25 days.

Case history: In late May, 1978, the girl suffered severe arthralgia in both knee joints which made it difficult for her to walk. A few days later, her left hand lost the ability to hold things due to its increasingly serious involuntary movement. Twenty days later, the involuntary movement affected all the limbs. By then, she had lost the ability to manage her own affairs, like putting on clothes and using chopsticks. The movement was so serious that it was even difficult to keep the blanket over her in place during night.

Physical examination: The patient had a clear state of mind; her speech was quick and inarticulate. She could not sit still and her eyes, eyebrows and limbs always moved automatically. The muscle tonus was reduced, but the pathological reflexes were negative. The heart beat was normal, 84 per minutes, and no valvular murmur was detected of the heart. The RBC sediment rate was 31 mm/hour and the WBC count was 10,700/cubic mm with 73 percent of neutrophils.

Selected stimulating area: Chorea and tremor controlling areas on both sides.

Treatment: Scalp acupuncture was applied once a day. After the first round of treatment, the involuntary movement of the limbs is somewhat relieved. After the third round, it markedly improved. After the fourth round, the involuntary movement of the right arm and leg stopped basically and the patient was able to comb hair, put on clothes and eat her own meal. The RBC sediment rate reduced to 5 mm/hour and the WBC count reduced to 6,500/cubic mm with 73 percent of neutrophils.

(2) Hemichorea

Hemichorea refers to involuntary choreic movement that is limited to limbs on one side of the body. It can either be chorea rheumatism or progressive chronic chorea. Besides, it may be the result of damage to the basal ganglia. Most of the patients are middle-aged and old people.

Selected stimulating area: Chorea and tremor controlling area on the opposite side of the symptoms.

Treatment: Scalp acupuncture, applied once a day, can greatly relieve the symptoms. Some patients may be cured after a period of treatment.

Case Report:

(1) Right hemichorea

Wang, male, 58 years old, from Yuncheng, Shanxi Province.

Chief complaint: Involuntary movement in the right limbs for three days.

Case history: On the morning of August 19, 1978, the patient found he could not hold a basin because of the swaying movement of his right hand. Shortly after, the whole right arm and right leg were affected.

Physical examination: The patient had a sober mind and normal speech. The right nasolabial groove was shallower than the left one. The muscular strength of both hands was normal and each had a gripping strength of 28 kg. The gait was not steady and even. The pathological reflexes were negative.

Now and then, the right forearm adducted and supinated involuntarily and the fingers suddenly flexed slightly, about 26 times per minute. The right knee frequently adducted over a range of 10 centimetres. The blood pressure was 168/80 mmHg and the heart beat was regular, 82 per minutes. No valvular murmur of the heart was detected, and the ECG was normal.

Selected stimulating area: Chorea and tremor controlling area on the left side.

Treatment: Scalp acupuncture was applied once a day. After the first round of treatment, the involuntary movement of the right limbs was relieved. On the same night, the patient only felt the involuntary twitching in the right limbs while other people could not see it. The next morning, the patient's feeling of the abnormal twitching also disappeared. The choreic movement was entirely stopped after 10 rounds of treatment.

(2) Right hemichorea with slight hemiplegia of right limbs

Yang, female, 71 years old, from Linyi County, Shanxi Province.

Chief complaint: Weakness and involuntary movement of right limbs for four and half months.

Case history: One day in November 1978, the patient found that her right hand was so weak that it could not hold any thing and the movement of her right leg was impaired. Since February 15, 1979, her right limbs were caught in involuntary and uncontrollable movement.

Physical examination: The blood pressure was 180/90 mmHg and the heart beat was 80 per minutes. She was sober-minded. The involuntary movement of the right limbs could not be controlled when she tried to sit still on a chair. Both arms could move within the normal range, although the muscular strength of the right arm was weak. The Hoffmann's sign was negative.

Diagnosis: Right hemichorea.

Selected stimulating areas: Left chorea and tremor controlling area, and upper three-fifths of left motor area and left motor and sensory area of foot.

Treatment: Scalp acupuncture was applied once a day. After five rounds of treatment, the involuntary movement of the right limbs was obviously controlled. After 15 rounds of treatment, the involuntary movement of the right arm completely disappeared except some tremors in the right foot. The patient could walk independently. The patient was entirely cured after 21 rounds of treatment.

(3) Progressive Chronic Chorea (Huntington's Chorea)

Progressive chronic chorea is a hereditary disease with a slow progression of choreic movement and dementia due to changes in basal ganglia and cerebral cortex.

A rare disease, it is more common in people between 35 and 40 years old. The symptoms appear when people are 20-50 years old. It is a typical dominant inheritant disease of chromosome and the morbidity rate is 50 percent for each generation in both sexes.

Autopsy shows that the caudate and putamen nuclei are mostly affected.

The most important symptoms of the disease are choreic movement along with dementia. At the early stage, the patients are found to just have awkward movement and unsteadiness as well as some involuntary movement, such as shrugging the shoulders, twitching the fingers and "making faces." The choreic movement may gradually become worse and worse, with the muscles of face, trunk and limbs all affected.

Selected stimulating areas: Chorea and tremor controlling areas on both sides.

Treatment: Scalp acupuncture, applied once a day, may relieve the symptoms in some patients.

Case Report:

Han, male, 49 years old, from Fuxin City, Liaoning Province.

Chief complaint: Involuntary movement of all limbs for over two years.

Case history: More than two years before, the movement of the patient's limbs became abnormally quicker than usual. At first, he himself and his family did not consider it a disease. Half a year later, the condition became worse—his hands could not hold things firmly and he often knitted his eyebrows and winked eyes unintentionally. A year later, the choreic movement affected his legs which made it difficult for him to walk steadily. Routine acupuncture as well as Western and traditional therapies failed to stop the progress of the disease.

Physical examination: The patient had a clear state of mind and had a quick speech and an irritable mood. He constantly knitted eyebrows, winked eyes and moved limbs involuntarily. He had a unsteady and faltering gait. When sleeping at night, the blanket could not be kept safely in place because of the violent involuntary movement of his limbs. He had difficulty in putting on clothes by himself. He could not use chopsticks to pick up food, and the bread he held in hand frequently dropped down when eating. He also had difficulty to write and to pick up things.

Selected stimulating areas: Chorea and tremor controlling areas on both sides.

Treatment: Scalp acupuncture was applied once a day. After treatment, the frequency of the choreic movement reduced and the patient could sleep with the blanket safely covered over his body. After 20 rounds of treatment, the involuntary movement of the limbs was much controlled and it almost stopped when he was quiet. The patient could finish a meal without dropping the chopsticks or bread and his handwriting was much improved.

2. Paralysis Agitans

Paralysis agitans, also called Parkinson's disease, is a degenerative disease of the central nervous system, with the lesions mainly lying in the substantia nigra and corpus striatum. The disease usually occurs among middle-aged people. Its major symptoms are tremor, muscular spasm and reduced action.

(1) Tremor

Tremor is the most symptom of this disease. At the early stage, light tremor will appear only when the patient is nervous, and it will disappear when the patient is calmed down. Such a condition may last over a long period of time. During this period, a wrong diagnosis may be made that the patient has contracted neurasthenia. At the second stage, the tremor will appear when the patient is calm and it will temporarily stop when the patient does something. At the late stage, it will always be there even when the patient does something. Moreover, it can get more serious when the patient undergoes an emotional disturbance. However, it stops completely during sleep or under anaesthesia.

(2) Slow motion and reduced action. Slow motion and reduced action are due to the increase of muscular tonus and a series of motor disturbances in posture maintenance and balance reflex. At the early stage, only such delicate movement like writing is affected and the patient often shows a "hurrying" gait and a "mask" face; and at the late stage, he or she will not be able to walk at all.

In the clinical practice, the author and his colleagues have observed that motor disturbance can be temporarily relieved for two or three hours by scalp acupuncture. This may provide an additional clue for further studying the pathogenesis of this disease.

(3) Increase of muscular tonus: The increase of muscular tonus is due to damage of the extrapyramidal system. It can be divided into the lead-pipe rigidity and cogwheel rigidity. In the former, the muscular tonus and the resistance to passive movement are maintained evenly. But in the latter, a rhythmical change of resistance with an intermittent pause of movement can be induced with a cogwheel sensation when the limb is passively moved. Some patients may have an impaired sensation.

The disease, along with its above-mentioned symptoms, if caused by cerebral arteriosclerosis, CO intoxication or cerebral injury, is called Parkinson's syndrome.

Selected stimulating area: Chorea and tremor controlling area as the first choice.

Treatment: Scalp acupuncture is applied once a day at the selected stimulating area on both sides if the symptoms appear on both sides of the body. Otherwise, it is applied at the selected stimulating area on the side opposite to the symptoms. For patients who only show the symptoms of slow motion and reduced action, scalp acupuncture should be applied at the motor areas on both sides; and for patients who also have the impaired sensation, the sensory area should be added for treatment. Scalp acupuncture can relieve the symptoms of some patients. In a few cases, it can made the symptoms disappear.

Case Report:
(1) Parkinson's disease
Zhang, male, 42 years old, from Wuhan, Hubei Province.
Chief complaint: Tremor in all limbs for more than two years.
Case history: Two and a half years before, the patient developed dizziness, stiff neck, insomnia and unsteady gait. A diagnosis of neurasthenia was made by the local physician. So, he was treated with sedatives and glutamic acid without any

effect. Half a year later, mild tremor appeared in his left leg, accompanied by slow motion and reduced step length in walking. In August 1974, the tremor also affected both his hands. Then, a diagnosis of Parkinson's disease was made and he was treated with Artane, 1 mg each time and three times a day. But, the treatment was discontinued nine days later because of the intolerable side effects of dizziness, blurred vision, stomach upset and vomiting and also because of the ineffectiveness of the drug. Then, Levodopa was administered from half a pill to two and a half pills each time and three times a day for half a year. During the period when the medicine was administered, the symptoms were slightly relieved. All of a sudden, one day his arms and legs lost the ability to move.

Physical examination: The patient had a sober mind and a slightly dull facial expression; he had difficulty to turn his head and saliva dropped out of his mouth. He had tremor in all limbs while sitting still and walked at a typical "hurrying" gait, with difficulty to quickly stop and change direction. The muscular tonus increased with cogwheel rigidity.

Selected stimulating area: Chorea and tremor controlling area on both sides.

Treatment: After the first round of treatment by scalp acupuncture, the patient felt his neck was much more flexible and his mind became much clearer. He could straighten his back, walk in bigger strides and change direction easily. Yet, this condition existed for only three hours and all the symptoms returned. Altogether, 30 rounds of treatment by scalp acupuncture were given and each round produced a similar spell of relief. To lengthen the interval of relief, the needle-embedding method was tried out, with the same result.

From his experience, the patient felt the therapeutic result was closely related to the skill to manipulate the needles as well as the emotional status of the patient. For instance, the author observed that one round of the treatment did not produce any effect because the patient was upset by a letter containing bad news from his family.

(2) Parkinson's disease

Ruth, female, university professor from California, U.S.A.

Chief complaint: Impaired movement of all limbs and difficulty to write for three years.

Case history: Not recorded. But she had been treated with various methods in the United States without any effect. She made a special trip to China for treatment by scalp acupuncture.

Physical examination: She had a sober mind. The movement of all limbs was impaired, so she had difficulty to write. The increase of muscular tonus with cogwheel rigidity was observed.

Treatment: After three rounds of treatment by scalp acupuncture, the symptoms were somewhat relieved, and after 20 rounds of treatment, the movement of the limbs was markedly improved and her handwriting became basically normal.

(3) Parkinson's disease

Sayelhanov, male, 65 years old, from Kirgizstan.

Chief complaint: Tremors in left arm and leg for 8 years.

Case history: Eight years before, the patient developed tremor in his left limbs without any apparent reason. The tremor was more serious when he was nervous. Many therapies had been tried to no avail.

Physical examination: The patient had a clear state of mind. The movement of his left leg was somewhat impaired and the tremor in his left hand continued when he sat still. Yet, the tremor of the hand became less apparent when he did something. The muscular tonus was increased with cogwheel rigidity.

Diagnosis: Parkinson's disease.

Selected stimulating area: Right chorea and tremor controlling area.

Treatment: Scalp acupuncture was applied once a day. After the second round of treatment, the tremor of the left hand became less frequent and spell of tremor shortened. After the tenth round of treatment, the strength of the left leg restored and the patient could walk at ease, and his handwriting became normal. The following letter was written by him in seemingly normal handwriting afterwards.

"From 1984, I began to suffer tremor in my left limbs. I had tried many therapies, including medical massage, acupuncture and various drugs, but none was a success. Although the treatment with 'HAKOM' produced some improvement, I still suffered from severe tremor and had difficulty to move. After treatment with scalp acupuncture by Mr. Jiao, my muscles were much relaxed and the tremor in my hand virtually disappeared. I'm overjoyed and would like to express my heartfelt thanks to him for the excellent therapeutic result."

3. Torsional Spasm

Torsional spasm is also called torsional or deformative dystonia characterized by disturbance of muscular tonus and violent involuntary torsion of the trunk and limbs. It can be divided into idiopathic type and symptomatic type that appear in patients of infection, vascular diseases, intoxication and tumours. Its unique symptoms are involuntary torsional movement and spasm of the head, neck, trunk, pelvis and limbs.

Selected stimulating area: Chorea and tremor controlling area on both sides.

Treatment: In some cases, scalp acupuncture can cure torsion spasm caused by intoxication.

Case Report: Torsional Spasm Caused by Haloperidol

Zhang, male, 18 years old, from Yuncheng, Shanxi Province.

Chief complaint: Involuntary torsion of the whole body for half a day.

Case history: Two months ago, the patient developed insomnia and headache because of nervousness. A hospital diagnosed his case as neurosis and prescribed haloperidol for him. After taking the medicine for the third time, he developed a painful feeling in the back, which later developed into torsional spasm of the head and body to the left side.

Physical examination: The patient had a clear state of mind but an abnormal facial expression due to forced spasm. The head passively turned to the left side for 100 degrees; the right arm and the trunk also twisted intermittently to the left side for a spell of 30 seconds to two minutes with an interval of several minutes in between. When the attack came, the patient perspired over the head. The muscular tonus went up in the right arm along with a slight cogwheel rigidity.

Selected stimulating area: Upper half of chorea and tremor controlling area on both sides.

Treatment: Scalp acupuncture was applied once a day. After the first round of treatment, the severity of the torsional movement was apparently relieved and the interval between the attacks lengthened to more than 10 minutes. The next morning, the patient was almost normal except the increase of muscular tonus with cogwheel rigidity. After the second round of treatment, he fully recovered.

V. Diseases of Peripheral Nerves

1. Facial Paralysis (Bell's Palsy)

Facial paralysis, chiefly referring to Bell's palsy, is an acute disease caused by non-suppurative inflammation of the facial nerve in stylomastoid foramen.

Peripheral facial paralysis always occurs on one side of the face and seldom on both sides. Its onset is prompt. Usually, people may suddenly find they have contracted partial paralysis of the face in early morning. Prior to or during the early stage of the onset, people often feel a little pain in the ear and the mastoid or mandibular region.

In most cases of facial paralysis, both the upper and lower parts of the mimetic muscles are severely affected, giving rise to the manifestations of disappearance of frontal wrinkles, widening of palpebral fissure, difficulty for the eye to close, shallow nasolabial groove, ptosis of labial angle and deviation of mouth and eye.

Selected stimulating area: Lower two-fifths of motor area on both sides.

Treatment: Scalp acupuncture can be applied once a day after a correct diagnosis is made. In most cases, it can obtain a satisfactory result.

Of the 128 cases of facial paralysis treated with scalp acupuncture, 124 were cured, accounting for 96.87 percent; three were greatly relieved, accounting for 2.34 percent; and only in one case, scalp acupuncture did not produce any effect.

2. Herpes Zoster

Herpes zoster is an acute infectious disease affecting first the primary sensory neurons and skin related to them.

At the early stage of herpes zoster over the limbs and trunk, the patients usually feel a burning and pricking pain over the cutaneous area covering one or two somatomes innervated by the infected nerve roots along with a hypersensitivity to pain in the neighbouring region. Three or four days later, papules, characterized by segmental distribution, appear over the skin surface and then turn into clusters of vesicles over an erythematous background. Still a few days later, the vesicles gradually become shrivelled and change into crusts. Small scars may remain permanently over the skin after the crusts are peeled off. The local pain may remain for several weeks or a few months or even forever. The post-herpetic neuralgia is more common in old patients. Some patients may have cutaneous pruritus.

Selected stimulating areas: Sensory area, and motor and sensory area of foot on both sides.

Treatment: Scalp acupuncture may produce an effective cure to pain caused by herpes zoster.

Of a total of 185 cases of herpes zoster treated with scalp acupuncture, 117 were cured, accounting for 63.24 percent; 47 were greatly relieved, accounting for 25.4 percent; 14 were improved, accounting for 7.56 percent; and seven did not see any therapeutic effect, accounting for 3.78 percent.

3. Acute Infective Polyradiculoneuritis (Acute Infective Polyneuritis)

The cause of the disease is still unknown. It may have something to do with viral infection or autoimmune reaction. Anyway, it is an acute or subacute disease. Before its onset, about 80 percent of the patients have the symptoms of infection, particularly infection of the upper respiratory tract or the intestine, the body temperature is 37.5-38.5 degrees centigrade and the WBC count is 15,000/cubic mm. About 10 days after the onset of the disease, the examination of cerebrospinal fluid (CSF) may show a dissociation phenomenon between the content of protein and WBC count. The protein content in the CSF may increase to 50-500 mg% while the WBC count either remains normal or increases slightly. The abnormally increased protein content may begin coming down 4-6 weeks later. An important clinical manifestation of this disease is quickly developed flaccid paralysis of all limbs, usually starting from the lower limbs and spreading to the upper ones and being symmetrical in distribution, with the muscles at the proximal part of the limbs being more seriously affected in most patients. More than half of the patients also experience damage of the cranial nerves and a small number suffer from paralysis of the respiratory muscles.

Selected stimulating areas: Upper three-fifths of motor area, and motor and sensory area of foot on both sides.

Treatment: Early treatment with scalp acupuncture, applied once day, can be given to patients without paralysis of the respiratory muscles. The therapeutic result is better for patients with a short clinical course and without damage of the cranial nerves. But, it is not so satisfactory for patients with radiculoneuritis of the lumbar and sacral nerves.

Of the 52 cases of acute infective polyradiculoneuritis treated with scalp acupuncture, 25 were cured, accounting for 48.07 percent; 11 were greatly relieved, accounting for 21.15 percent; 14 were somewhat relieved, accounting for 26.92 percent; and two did not see any effect.

4. Neuralgia Sciatica

Neuralgia sciatica is common; it is a syndrome characterized by pain that spreads along the pathway of the sciatic nerve and its innervated area. Usually, it occurs after the local lesions along the course of this nerve and can be divided into the root type and trunk type.

The sciatic nerve comprises the nerve roots of L4-S3 spinal nerves and is distributed all over the lower limbs through the hip region. Therefore, the pain radiates from the lower back, the buttocks, the posterior side of the thigh and posteriolateral side of the legs to the lateral border of the feet. Tenderness can also be detected along this route. Walking, movement of the lower limbs and stretch of the sciatic nerve will make the pain more serious. The symptoms due to injury of the partial nerve root or nerve trunk can be detected, such as impaired sensation, reduced muscular strength and reduction or disappearance of tendon reflex in the ankle joints.

Selected stimulating areas: Upper two-fifths of sensory area, and motor and sensory area of foot on both sides.

Treatment: Scalp acupuncture, applied once a day, can cure part of the cases. Moreover, it has the advantage of producing a quick therapeutic result in some patients.

Of the 148 cases of neuralgia sciatica treated with scalp acupuncture, 68 were cured, accounting for 45.94 percent; 42 were greatly relieved, accounting for 28.37 percent; 24 were somewhat relieved, accounting for 16.21 percent; and 14 did not see any effect.

VI. Cortical Frequent Urination, Dysuria and Incontinence of Urine

The disturbance of urination, including frequent urination, dysuria and incontinence of urine, can be caused by the dysfunction of the paracentral lobule of brain due to arteriosclerosis, insufficient blood supply of the anterior cerebral artery or cerebral thrombosis. To distinguish it from urinary disturbance due to diseases of the urinary system, it is called here separately as "cortical frequent urination," "cortical dysuria" and "cortical incontinence of urine."

Selected stimulating area: Motor and sensory area of foot on both sides.

Treatment: Scalp acupuncture, applied once a day, produces a good therapeutic effect in the treatment of cortical disturbance of urination. In particular, it can produce a quick cure for cortical frequent urination. Some patients can be greatly relieved or completely cured by just one round of treatment.

Of the 48 cases of polyuria (frequent urination) treated with scalp acupuncture, 37 were cured, accounting for 77.10 percent; eight were greatly relieved, accounting for 16.7 percent; two were somewhat relieved, accounting for 4.2 percent; and one did not see any effect.

Case Report:
(1) Cortical frequent urination

Wang, male, 57 years old, Houma, Shanxi Province.

Chief complaint: Inflexibility of the right leg along with frequent urination for half a year.

Case history: Half a year before, the patient suddenly felt the movement of his right leg became inflexible and the urination became very frequent, once every 20 minutes during day and 5-6 times during night. Both traditional and Western medicine was tried without success.

Physical examination: The patient had a clear state of mind and the functions of the cranial nerves were normal. The muscular tonus of both arms was normal and the pathological signs were negative. The muscular strength of the right leg reduced with an apparent hemiplegic gait to walk. Funduscopic examination showed a sign of crossing of the arterioles and venules.

Selected stimulating area: Motor and sensory area of foot on both sides.

Treatment: Scalp acupuncture was applied once a day. After seven rounds of treatment, the urination was reduced to 7-8 times a day and the muscular strength of the right leg was greatly improved.

(2) Cortical incontinence of urine

Chen, female, 49 years old, from Yuncheng, Shanxi Province.

Chief complaint: Incontinence of urine for three days.

Case history: The patient had hypertension with dizziness for several years. Three days before, she suddenly developed urgent urination and incontinence of urine. She often wetted her trousers before reaching the toilet.

Treatment: After just one round of treatment with scalp acupuncture, the urgent urination and incontinence of urine entirely disappeared. Follow-up visit four months later showed her urination remained perfectly normal ever since the treatment.

(3) Mellitus insipidus

Babayeba, female, 52 years old, Kirghizstan.

Chief complaint: Excessive much water intake and polyuria for more than 30 years.

Case history: Since 1962, the patient began to drink too much water and, because of the excessive water intake, she developed polyuria. On average, she drank 20-22 litres of water every day and passed urine every 20-30 minutes. She had tried various therapies but none had cured her disease.

Physical examination: The patient had a clear state of mind and could accurately express herself. There were no positive neurological signs. The blood sugar content was normal and the sugar content in urine was OK. The patient was not pathologically lean in appearance.

Diagnosis: Mellitus insipidus.

Selected stimulating areas: Motor and sensory area of foot and reproductive area on both sides.

Treatment: Scalp acupuncture was applied once a day. After the first round of treatment, her water intake came down. After the fourth round, she drank only 6-7 litres of water every day and the number of urination also reduced. After the sixth round, the water intake was further reduced to 5 litres per day and the frequency of urination became normal.

VII. Headache

Headache is a common symptom. It may be caused by both diseases of the nervous system and diseases of the whole body. So, headache has many causes, and it is imperative to make a correct diagnosis before treatment is given.

Selected stimulating areas: For headache in the parietal region, upper two-fifths of the sensory area on both sides are selected; and for headache in the frontal and temporal region, lower two-fifths of the sensory area on the contralateral side are selected. Generally speaking, for pain on one side of the head, select the sensory area on the opposite side, and for pain on both sides of the head, select the sensory area on both sides.

Treatment: Scalp acupuncture, applied once a day, can relieve angioneurotic headache, migraine and headache due to common cold in some patients.

Of the 463 cases of headache treated with scalp acupuncture, 236 were cured, accounting for 50.97 percent; 65 were greatly relieved, accounting for 14.03 percent; 134 were somewhat relieved, accounting for 28.94 percent; and 28 did not see any effect at all, accounting for 6.04 percent.

VIII. Hypertension

The etiology of hypertension is still uncertain. It is characterized by elevation of arterial blood pressure and can be a disease reflecting the pathological changes in the blood vessels, heart, brain and kidney.

All adults who have a blood pressure higher than 160/95 mmHg should be considered patients of hypertension, and those who have a blood pressure between 160/95 mmHg and 140/90 mmHg should considered patients of "critical hypertension." Patients of "critical hypertension" should be carefully monitored.

Selected stimulating areas: Upper half of the vascular dilation and constriction area on both sides.

Treatment: Scalp acupuncture, applied once a day, can produce different therapeutic results for different types of hypertension. In a few cases, it can produce a marvellous therapeutic effect just by one round of treatment.

Of a total of 50 patients of hypertension treated with scalp acupuncture, 25 were greatly relieved, accounting for 50 percent; 23 were somewhat relieved, accounting for 46 percent; and two did not see any effect at all.

Case Report:

(1) Shao, male, 63 years old, from Jishan County, Shanxi Province.

The patient had a five-year history of hypertension along with dizziness and insomnia. His blood pressure was 170/100 mmHg.

Scalp acupuncture was applied at the upper half of the vascular dilation and constriction area on both sides. After the needles were inserted, they were not manipulated but made to remain in place for 30 minutes. The patient's blood pressure went down to 120/70 mmHg and he himself felt his sufferings were much relieved.

(2) Refractory hypertension

Tuatpov, male, 58 years old, from Kirghizstan.

The patient had suffered from refractory hypertension, which was as high as 210/160 mmHg, for more than 10 years. He had tried many therapies and medicines without success. In April, 1993, he tried scalp acupuncture from the author in his country. Only after four rounds of treatment, his blood pressure went down to 160/100 mmHg. Record kept in the following 20-odd days showed that his blood pressure remained fairly stable (see Table 3-1).

**Table 3-1 Record of the Patient's Blood Pressure
After Scalp Acupuncture Treatment**

Date (1993)	Blood pressure (mmHg)
April 22	200/140
April 23	200/130
April 24	170/120
April 26	180/110
April 27	160/100
April 28	160/100
April 29	170/90
May 7	160/100
May 8	160/100
May 10	160/100
May 11	170/100
May 12	160/100
May 13	170/100
May 14	145/85
May 15	140/100

Section 2 Medical Diseases

I. Diseases of Respiratory System

1. Common Cold

Common cold is caused by rhinovirus in adults and by parainfluenza virus and respiratory syncytial virus in children. The incubation period of the disease is short, about one day, and its onset is prompt. At the early stage, patients develop a rough and dry sensation and pain in the throat, which are accompanied by sneezing, nasal obstruction and running nose. Later, the larynx, trachea and bronchi may be affected and thus the symptoms of hoarse voice, cough and pain in chest appear.

Selected stimulating areas: Thoracic cavity area and upper two-fifths of sensory area on both sides.

Treatment: Scalp acupuncture, applied once a day, can relieve the symptoms in some patients.

Case Report:

An, 50 years old, from Linfen, Shanxi Province.

Chief complaint: Chest pain, cough and shortness of breath after inflection of the upper respiratory tract for 7 days.

Case history: On November 1, 1977, the patient felt nasal obstruction. On the next day, he had running nose, stuffy feeling in the head, cough, short and difficult breathing, distension and discomfort in both sides of the chest as well as serious pain in the breast and back.

Selected stimulating areas: Thoracic cavity area and upper two-fifths of sensory area on both sides.

Treatment: When the needles were inserted in place, the patient felt a distending sensation and relief in the shortness of breath. A hot sensation was produced in the chest and back by quick manipulation of the needles. After the needles were manipulated for three rounds, pain and discomfort in chest and back were completely gone, his breathing returned to normal and he felt refreshed in the head and eyes. The patient was completely cured after the second round of treatment the next day.

2. Bronchial Asthma

Bronchial asthma is a common allergic disease of the lungs with seasonal attacks. When it attacks, the patients may suffer from chest distress, shortness of breath, wheezing noise in the throat and cough with sputum due to spasm of the smooth muscle of the bronchioles and congestion, edema and increase of secretion of the respiratory mucosa. It may be caused by the inhalation of antigen particles or the infection of respiratory tract.

Usually, there are some prodromal symptoms before the onset of the disease, such as the cough, chest distress or repeated sneezing. These symptoms, if not timely treated, will quickly develop into asthma. In acute cases, the patients suffer from shortness of breath, wheezing noise in the throat and cough with much sputum, and wheezing rales can be heard in the lungs by auscultation.

Selected stimulating area: Thoracic cavity area on both sides.

Treatment: Scalp acupuncture, applied once a day, can relieve the symptoms in some patients.

Of the 209 cases of bronchial asthma we treated with scalp acupuncture, 83 were cured, accounting for 39.71 percent; 93 were greatly relieved, accounting for 44.49 percent; 28 were some improved, accounting for 13.39 percent; and five did not see any effect at all.

Case Report:

(1) Bronchial asthma

Wang, female, two years old, from Yuncheng, Shanxi Province.

Case history: Two days before, the girl began to have cough, fever and asthma. Although the fever was relieved by the administration of antipyretic, asthma and shortness of breath continued.

Physical examination: The patient had a clear state of mind and obvious asthma. Wheezing rales could be detected in both lungs.

Selected stimulating area: Thoracic cavity area on both sides.

Treatment: Scalp acupuncture was applied once a day. Five minutes after the insertion of needles in the first round of treatment, the asthma was somewhat relieved and 30 minutes later it completely stopped. The wheezing rales in the lungs also disappeared. After nine rounds of treatment, the asthma had never recurred.

(2) Allergic dyspnea

Wu, female, 32 years old, from Jiangxian County, Shanxi Province.

Chief complaint: Dyspnea and shortness of breath for over four years.

Case history: Four years before, the patient developed shortness of breath after an attack of common cold and the sufferings regularly reappeared due to the change of weather or the inhalation of some drugs, such as the lysol. Each spell of attack might last for several months.

Physical examination: The patient showed a clear state of mind and took a thoracic respiration with much effort. The breathing was rough, but without wheezing noise in the lungs.

Selected stimulating area: Thoracic cavity area on both sides.

Treatment: After needles were embedded for three hours, the shortness of breath was apparently relieved. On the second day, the thoracic respiration disappeared and the breathing became normal. The treatment continued for 12 days before the patient completely recovered.

II. Male Sexual Disorders

The sexual disorders of males can be divided into the organic and functional types. The latter is more common and can be again divided into two subtypes: One is due to disturbance of the cerebral cortex and the other is due to disturbance of the nerve reflexes. Sexual disorders of the former subtype are caused by anxiety and misgivings about sexual activity or due to memory of failures in past sexual life; while in those of the latter subtype, the nerve reflexes of sexual activity are inhibited by long-term mental depression because of one's own sexual desire cannot be satisfied.

In clinical practice, sexual disorders can be divided into those due to over excitement of sexual reflexes, such as emission and premature seminal ejaculation, and those due to excessive inhibition of sexual reflexes, such as impotence.

Emission refers to seminal discharge without sexual intercourse, premature ejaculation means early seminal discharge before the process of sexual intercourse finishes, and impotence suggests failure of erection of the penis to carry out normal sexual activity.

Selected stimulating areas: Motor and sensory area of foot and reproductive area on both sides.

Treatment: Scalp acupuncture, applied once a day, can produce a satisfactory therapeutic effect in most of the cases.

Of a total of 110 cases of impotence treated with scalp acupuncture, eight were cured, accounting for 7.3 percent; 59 were greatly relieved, accounting for 53.6 percent; 21 were relieved by lesser degrees, accounting for 19.1 percent; and 22 did not show any effect at all, accounting for 20 percent.

Case Report:

(1) Emission

Lin, 25 years old, from Yuncheng, Shanxi Province.

Chief complaint: Emission for more than six years.

Case history: Six years before, the patient got the habit of masturbation. By and by, he developed night emission along with dreams of sexual intercourse once every two or three days. The emission continued after marriage and became worse, which made him very nervous. He had various both traditional Chinese medicine and Western medicine without much success. So, he came to the hospital for treatment with scalp acupuncture.

Selected stimulating areas: Motor and sensory area of foot and reproductive area on both sides.

Treatment: Scalp acupuncture was applied once a day. During the treatment, he had only two emissions, after the first and fifth round of treatment respectively. Since then, he had no more emission for 24 days in succession. Moreover, he felt he was energetic throughout the day.

(2) Impotence and premature ejaculation

Zhang, 26 years old, from Yuncheng, Shanxi Province.

Chief complaint: Impotence and premature ejaculation for half a year.

Case history: Half a year before, the patient experienced two emissions at night because fatigue. He became very nervous and gradually developed insomnia, impotence, premature ejaculation and loss of sexual appetite. He was very much worried as his wife asked for a divorce because of the unsatisfied sexual life between husband and wife. Under such mental pressure, his penis even shrank and retracted, to say nothing of getting erected during the sexual intercourse.

Selected stimulating areas: Motor and sensory area of foot and reproductive area on both sides.

Treatment: Scalp acupuncture was applied once a day. After the first round of treatment, the patient was able to sleep well at night with the penis getting erected occasionally. After seven rounds of treatment, the sexual intercourse and seminal ejaculation returned to normal.

(3) Impotence

Zhang, from Taiyuan, Shanxi Province.

Chief complaint: Impotence for one year and half.

Case history: After an operation for stomach perforation in 1978, the patient lost his sexual desire completely and his penis could not get erected for love-making.

Selected stimulating areas: Motor and sensory area of foot and reproductive area on both sides.

Treatment: Scalp acupuncture was applied once a day. After five rounds of treatment, the patient's penis could occasionally erect. After the eighth round of treatment, it could erect more frequently at night and the patient's sexual desire returned. Follow-up visit a month's later proved the therapeutic result to be satisfactory.

III. Diarrhoea

Diarrhoea is clinically common. It refers to increased bowel movements to pass thin stool or stool with pus and blood.

Selected stimulating areas: Motor and sensory area of foot and reproductive area on both sides.

Treatment: Scalp acupuncture, applied once a day, can stop diarrhoea in some cases.

Case Report:

(1) Ge, female, 63 years old, Yuncheng, Shanxi Province.

Chief complaint: Abdominal pain and diarrhoea for more than one year.

Case history: One year before, the patient developed abdominal pain in early morning, followed by bowel movement to pass thin stool each day. She also suffered from insomnia, poor appetite and low spirit. She had tried other therapies without success and was admitted on June 9, 1978.

Diagnosis: Early morning diarrhoea.

Selected stimulating areas: Motor and sensory area of foot and reproductive area on both sides.

Treatment: Scalp acupuncture was applied once a day. After three rounds of treatment, the abdominal pain in early morning was relieved, but the diarrhoea remained. After the fourth round, the abdominal pain and diarrhoea were both controlled. The disease was completely cured after treatment for 10 days.

On June 29, 1978, the abdominal pain and diarrhoea recurred, but the disease was again controlled by the intermittent treatment with scalp acupuncture for one month.

(2) Jia, male, 60 years old, from Yuncheng, Shanxi Province.

Chief complaint: Abdominal pain and diarrhoea for four months.

Case history: On may 16, 1978, the patient began to have stool with pus and blood, 14-15 times a day, which could not be controlled by routine Western and traditional Chinese medicine. The disease became more serious since September 26, 1978 when the patient passed bloody stool for 15-16 times on average in daytime and one or two times at night.

Selected stimulating areas: Motor and sensory area of foot and reproductive area on both sides.

Treatment: Scalp acupuncture was applied once a day. After the first round of treatment, abdominal distension disappeared and bowel movement, without pus and blood, reduced to 5-6 times a day on the second day. After the fourth round of treatment, bowel movement further reduced to four times. What was left was only some abdominal distension. After the treatment on the fifth day, he had only one bowl movement and abdominal distension disappeared. The therapeutic result was proved by follow-up visit 50 days later.

IV. Diabetes Mellitus

Diabetes mellitus is a common metabolic and endocrinal disease, perhaps with a hereditary cause, and its etiology is still unknown. The fundamental pathophysiological change is the metabolic disturbance regarding carbohydrate, fat and protein due to absolute or relative deficiency of insulin. Characterized by the increase of blood and urine sugar, its has such basic clinical manifestations as polyuria, increased water and food intake, fatigue and pathological emaciation. In severe cases, the patients may develop ketoacidosis.

In terms of age brackets, the diabetes mellitus patients can be divided into the juvenile group and the adult group, and in terms of severity of the disease, they can be divided into mild cases, moderately severe cases and severe cases.

(a) Mild cases: There were not clinical manifestations; the blood sugar is below 150 mg%; and people are only found to have contracted the disease in routine physical checks or after they have suffered from some sort of infection.

(b) Moderately severe cases: Those cases with clinical manifestations between the mild and severe cases.

(c) Severe cases: The patients are relatively young or have been sick for quite some time and show apparent pathological emaciation. The blood sugar, tested when the stomach is empty, is often higher than 250 mg%.

Selected stimulating areas: Motor and sensory area of foot and reproductive area on both sides.

Treatment: Scalp acupuncture, applied once a day at the selected stimulating areas, can produce certain therapeutic effect to reduce polyuria and increased intake of water.

Case Report:

Xu, female, 53 years old, from Yuncheng, Shanxi Province.

Chief complaint: Polydipsia, increased intake of water, polyuria and pathological emaciation for more than five years.

Case history: Without any obvious reason, the patient began to have increased water and food intake, polyuria, hunger and polydipsia five years before. She took 8-10 litres of water on average per day and always had a desire of urination and passed urine one or two times every hour and 7-8 times at night. Despite the large meals she had, the patient became increasingly emaciated. Her urine sugar was positive (++++). She had tried in succession D860, phenformin and patent herbal drugs without much effect. On the contrary, she gradually developed abdominal distension, arthralgia, blurred vision and insomnia.

Physical examination: The patient had a clear state of mind, and a pale complexion and emaciated physique. Her weight was only 48 kg. The heart beat was regular, without valvular murmur, and the pulse beat was 84 per minute. The lungs were clear without rales; the liver and spleen were not palpable. Funduscopic examination showed patches of waxy infiltration. Pitting edema was found over the front aspect of both tibia bones. The urine sugar was positive (+++).

Diagnosis: Diabetes mellitus.

Selected stimulating areas: Motor and sensory area of foot and reproductive area on both sides.

Treatment: The scalp acupuncture was applied once a day. After two rounds of treatment, the patient's spirit, sleep and vision were improved and her water intake and urine discharge were reduced. After seven rounds of treatment, her spirit was even better, her water intake was reduced to 1.5 litre, and her urination was reduced to seven times a day. After 10 rounds of treatment, the abdominal distension was relieved, the pitting edema over both legs disappeared, and the sensation of hunger and amount of food intake were controlled. And after 20 rounds of treatment, her body weight went up to 51.5 kg, the intake of staple food and water was reduced to 500 g and 1.5 litre respectively each day, but the urine sugar was still positive (+++). The therapeutic result was consolidated by another 50 rounds of treatment.

Section 3 External Diseases

I. Bone Diseases

(1) Cervical Hypertrophic Osteoarthropathy

Cervical hypertrophic osteoarthropathy, also called cervical spondylopathy, is a common ailment of the cervical spine, with the pathological change in the cervical vertebrae, intervertebral discs and their surrounding connective tissues as well as the degeneration of spinal nerve roots and spinal cord. The major symptoms are pain in the head, neck, arm, hand and chest, and progressive disturbance of sensation and movement of the limbs. Severe cases may develop into paraplegia. This disease is seen more often in adults between 40 and 60 years old.

X-ray pictures of the cervical spine may show the narrowing of the intervertebral space and the formation of labial osteophyte along the anterior and posterior sides of the vertebral body.

Selected stimulating areas: Motor and sensory area of foot and upper two-fifths of the sensory area on the opposite side of the symptoms and on both sides for with symptoms on both sides.

Treatment: Scalp acupuncture, applied once a day, can greatly relieve the clinical manifestations in some patients.

Case Report:

Shi, male, 58 years old, from Yuncheng, Shanxi Province.

Chief complaint: Numbness in left arm for nine months and in right arm for four months.

Case history: In August 1977, the patient developed numbness in the left arm without any apparent reason. The severity of the numbness gradually became more serious. In January 1978, he felt pain in the right arm when the arm was swayed forward and backward or abducted. The patient could not sleep well at night because he would have pain in the arm lying on either side. Sometimes, he even could not walk for severe pain in both legs. Treatment with ordinary acupuncture, physical therapy and injection of testosterone propionate all failed to relieve the sufferings.

Physical examination: The patient had a clear state of mind and could clearly express himself. A belt-like pain-reduction zone, 0.5 centimetre in width, was found stretching from the side of the fifth cervical vertebra to the left shoulder, the posterior mid-line of the upper arm and the lateral border of the forearm, the thumb and index finger. The reduction of the pain sensation in this zone was proved by pricking test with a pin. The patient had serious pain over the deltoid muscle and the lateral region of the clavicle when moving the right arm. The right elbow joint would be in great pain when flexed. The patient could not take things out of the coat pocket and raise the arm when lying in a sling chair. He always kept his chin down and the elbow joint flexed and fixed when walking. X-ray pictures showed labial osteophyte along the anterior and posterior borders of the third to the seventh cervical vertebrae.

Selected stimulating area: Motor and sensory area of foot on both sides.

Treatment: Scalp acupuncture was applied once a day. The numbness and pain in both arms disappeared right after the first treatment, but returned the same night. Hence, the needle-embedding method was adopted to consolidate the therapeutic result. All together, 50 rounds of treatment were given. After the treatment, all clinical symptoms and physical signs completely disappeared and the patient went back to work. A follow-up visit eight months later showed he was in perfect health.

(2) Lumbar Hypertrophic Osteoarhropathy

This disease, also called lumbar spinal canal stenosis or cauda equina claudication, is due to the congenital stenosis of the lumbar and sacral spinal canal and the hyperosteogeny of sacral vertebrae and their joints, which cause an impairment of blood supply and compression to the nerve roots.

The onset and development of the disease is very insidious and slow. Most patients have a long history of pain in the back, waist and posterior part of the thigh, and the pain radiates to the anterior and lateral sides of both legs and is accompanied with numbness and abnormal sensation in those regions.

X-ray check-up of the lumbosacral spine may show an apparent narrowing of the spinal canal and osteophyte on the anterior and posterior borders of the vertebrae.

Selected stimulating areas: Motor and sensory area of foot and upper two-fifths of the sensory area on the opposite side of the symptoms and on both sides for patients with symptoms on both sides.

Treatment: Scalp acupuncture, applied once a day, can relieve the clinical manifestations in some patients.

Case Report:

Liu, female, 48 years old, from Yuncheng, Shanxi Province.

Chief complaint: Lumbago and pain in the legs for three years.

Case history: Three years before, that is, in July 1975, the patient developed pain in the lower back without any apparent cause. Then the pain spread to the legs. While lying on bed, the patient had to move the legs with her hands. Physical therapy and treatment with both Western and traditional drugs failed to cure the sufferings. The symptom became even more serious over the recent month or more when the patient could not turn over in bed or sit up from bed in the morning. In the daytime, the patient could not stand up from her sitting posture for the lumbago, and both walking and coughing could induce and increase the pain in the lumbar region and legs.

Physical examination: Forward bending of the waist caused apparent pain in the inguinal groove and cough caused pain in the waist and buttocks. X-ray check-up showed obvious osteophyte on the anterior and posterior borders of the second to fourth lumbar vertebrae.

Selected stimulating areas: Motor and sensory area of foot and upper two-fifths of the sensory area on both sides.

Treatment: Scalp acupuncture was applied once a day. After the first round of treatment, the patient felt much relaxed in the waist and legs and the pain in the waist did not appear when she turned over in bed at night and got up and walked in early morning. Neither did it occur when she bent over the waist for a long time. After five rounds of treatment, soreness also disappeared, and she could freely move the waist to all directions without pain. Follow-up visit two months later proved the therapeutic result.

(3) Occult Spina Bifida

Patients with this disorder constitute over 30 percent of all patients with spina bifida. Most of them do not show any clinical symptoms and are accidentally found to have contracted this disease by X-ray checks, and only a small number of them have local soreness and discomfort. In a tiny number of patients, the caudal nerves may be stuck to the sacral bone and the abnormal lipofibrotic tissue may penetrate into the spinal canal. Along with the increase of age, the cauda equina may gradually move upward to stretch or compress the affected nerves to produce some symptoms and damage the caudal nerves, giving rise to such manifestations as functional disturbance of the sphincter muscles, reduction of muscular strength and dystrophy of the distal part of lower limbs.

Selected stimulating areas: Motor and sensory area of foot and upper two-fifths of the sensory area on both sides.

Treatment: Scalp acupuncture, applied once a day, can relieve the symptoms in some patients.

Case Report:

Guo, male, 28 years old, from Yuncheng, Shanxi Province.

Chief complaint: Pain in the lumbar and sacral region for more than one year.

Cases history: More than one year before, the patient developed pain and discomfort in the lumbar and sacral region, which lasted for several days. The pain became much more serious in the recent two months before he came to seek scalp acupuncture treatment on July 11, 1978.

Physical examination: The patient could not stretch his back straight for pain in the lower part of the back, and the pain could be made more serious by coughing and bending the back. X-ray examination showed failure of fusion of the fifth lumbar and the first sacral vertebrae. The red blood cell sediment rate was 5 mm/hr.

Selected stimulating areas: Motor and sensory area of foot and upper two-fifths of the sensory area on both sides.

Treatment: Scalp acupuncture was applied once a day. After the two rounds of treatment, the lumbago was much relieved; and after the third round, the back could be stretched straight. When all 20 rounds of treatment were completed, pain had vanished and no pain was induced by coughing, bending the back, sitting, standing and walking in the lower back.

II. Dermatological Diseases

(1) Cutaneous Pruritus

Itching is a symptom rather than a disease. It can be divided into the local and general types. The cutaneous pruritus discussed is paroxysmal in nature, usually lasting for a few hours. It can be caused or made more serious by drinking or taking spicy food.

For most people, the itching is more serious in night time than during the day. Sometimes, it can be so severe that people cannot but scratch the skin continuously until blood oozes out of the skin and the itching is offset by pain. As a result, the skin is often covered with scratches, bloody marks and pigmentation.

Selected stimulating areas: Motor and sensory area of foot and upper two-fifths of the sensory area on both sides.

Treatment: Scalp acupuncture, applied once a day, can cure itching in some patients.

Case Report:

Xie, female, 50 years old, from Yuncheng, Shanxi Province.

Chief complaint: Itching all over the body for more than two years.

Case history: Two years before, without any apparent reason the patient developed itching all over the body. The itching was so severe that she could not go to sleep at night and continuously scratched the skin. Western and traditional Chinese medicine could only produce a temporary relief and she came to the hospital for help on June 21, 1978.

Physical examination: Areas covered with bloody crusts and pigmentation because of scratching were found in all limbs, the chest and the back.

Selected stimulating area: Motor and sensory area of foot and upper two-fifths of the sensory area on both sides.

Treatment: Scalp acupuncture was applied once a day. After the third round of treatment, itching was relieved; and after the ninth round, it disappeared completely.

(2) Contact Dermatitis

Contact dermatitis refers to acute skin inflammation caused by contact with some irritative matters, including animals, plants or chemicals. The major manifestations are erythema, swelling, vesicles and bullae with itching and a burning sensation.

Selected stimulating areas: Motor and sensory area of foot and upper three-fifths of the sensory area on the opposite side of the lesions, or on both sides if the lesions are found on both sides of the body.

Treatment: Scalp acupuncture, applied once a day, can produce a cure for some patients.

Case Report:

Niu, female, 53 years old, from Qingxu County, Shanxi Province.

Chief complaint: Redness, swelling, eruption and itching in both hands for six days.

Case history: Six days before, red and itching rashes appeared over the face and in the dorsum of both hands without any apparent reason. Because of the severe itching produced by the rashes, the patient kept scratching her face and the dorsum of her hands.

Treatment: After manipulating the needles the first time, the itching disappeared; and after manipulating them for three rounds, the patient had a comfortable feeling all over the body. The redness, itching and swelling in the face and hands all disappeared the next day. Three more rounds of treatment were given to consolidate the therapeutic effect.

(3) Neurodermatitis

Neurodermatitis is a chronic dermatitis characterized by local itching and thickened skin, deepened sulci and polygonal papules. Two types—local and disseminated—are more common.

Selected stimulating areas: Motor and sensory area of foot and upper three-fifths of the sensory area on the opposite side of the lesions; and for lesions that appear on both sides, select the above areas on both sides.

Treatment: Scalp acupuncture, applied once a day, can cure the lesions in some patients.

Case Report:

Ran, female, 46 years old, from Yuncheng, Shanxi Province.

Chief complaint: Itching and roughness of skin over the radial side of both wrists for one and half a year.

Case history: In March 1977, the patient developed itching in both wrists without any apparent reason. The itching was so serious that the patient could not sleep at night. Later, the skin around the wrists gradually turned rough. Later, it spread to the neck, the inner thighs and chest. By the time she came to the hospital, she had itching all over the body.

Physical examination: The patient had a clear state of mind and could clearly express herself. The rough skin bulged over the normal skin with deep sulci and bloody crust. They were found in bilateral inguinal grooves and were 22×8 cm in size; in areas lateral and below both breasts, 8×6 cm; in popliteal fossae, 4×3 cm; and on the radial side of the palms and wrists, 12×12 cm. There were polygonal papules in some areas.

Selected stimulating areas: Motor and sensory area of foot and upper two-fifths of sensory area on both sides.

Treatment: Scalp acupuncture was applied once a day. After the third round of treatment, the general itching was markedly relieved, the skin lesions over both wrists were reduced to 6×6 cm in size and the lesions over other areas were also reduced in size. After 31 rounds of treatment, all skin lesions almost disappeared, leaving just some dark brown pigmentation patches and minimal local itching. And after 40 rounds of treatment, the itching was entirely gone.

(4) Alopecia Areata

Alopecia areata is a skin disease characterized by sudden and local loss of hair. But in severe cases, all the patients' hair may be lost. Usually, it is caused by mental trauma and emotional disturbance.

At the beginning, the hair falls out in round or oval-shaped patches 1-2 centimetres in size and with clearly seen boundaries. These patches will combine together as their number increases. In more serious cases, all the hair may fall, while the skin of the scalp will look normal and smooth, giving no sign of infection.

Selected stimulating areas: Motor and sensory area of foot and upper three-fifths of sensory area on both sides.

Treatment: Scalp acupuncture, applied once a day, can make hair to grow again in some patients.

Of a total of 67 patients of alopecia treated with scalp acupuncture, 47 were cured, accounting for 70.14 percent; 16 were markedly relieved, accounting for 23.88 percent; and four did not see any effect at all.

Case Report:

Jin, male, 14 years old, from Jishan County, Shanxi Province.

Chief complaint: Complete loss of hair and eyebrows for over seven months.

Case history: In October 1974, the boy saw a snake in an underground case and was terribly frightened. A few days later, his hair fell out in patches. In about a month's time, he lost all hair and eyebrows. Various therapies, including oral administration of glutamic acid, washing with decoction of Cacumen Biotae and rubbing with raw ginger, did not succeed to bring the hair out. So, he came to the hospital on August 21, 1975.

Physical examination: All hair and eyebrows had fallen and he was completely bald.

Selected stimulating areas: Motor and sensory area of foot and sensory area on both sides.

Treatment: After 20 rounds of treatment, the hair began to grow again, but it was sparse and thin, and yellow in color. After 30 rounds of treatment, the hair became more profuse and turned black in color, but it was limited to the frontal and parietal region of the head. And after 80 rounds of treatment, the hair and eyebrows became basically normal in lustre and color.

Section 4 Diseases of Ear

(1) Meniere's Disease and Meniere's Syndrome

Caused by edema, inflammation, vascular spasm, bleeding, arteriosclerosis, etc., Meniere's syndrome is characterized by paroxysmal vertigo and the feeling of turning of things, along with nausea, vomiting, pale complexion, nystagmus and ataxia. Each attack may last several hours or a few days.

Selected stimulating area: Dizziness and auditory area on both sides.

Treatment: Scalp acupuncture, applied once a day, produces a better therapeutic effect in treating Meniere's syndrome than in treating Meniere's disease. In a few cases, the sufferings can be relieved immediately after the needles are inserted.

Of a total of 786 cases of Meniere's disease and Meniere's syndrome treated with scalp acupuncture, 426 were cured, accounting for 54.19 percent; 174 were markedly relieved, accounting for 22.13 percent; 167 were relieved at lesser degrees, accounting for 21.24 percent; and 19 did not show any effect. From these statistics, it can be concluded scalp acupuncture is quite effective in treating Meniere's disease and Meniere's syndrome.

Case Report:

Bai, female, 50 years old, from Yuncheng, Shanxi Province.

Chief complaint: Vertigo for five years, more serious in the recent year.

Case history: The patient began to suffer from paroxysmal vertigo five years before, along with a rotating sensation, palpitation and perspiration. There were several attacks a day, with each lasting 20 minutes and the longest, 20 hours. The patient was admitted on May 26, 1978.

Physical examination: Apparent vertigo and an obvious rotating sensation of things around, tinnitus, palpitation and perspiration.

Selected stimulating area: Dizziness and auditory area on both sides.

Treatment: Scalp acupuncture was applied once a day. Vertigo entirely disappeared after the second round of treatment. There was a relapse five months later, which was cured again by scalp acupuncture.

(2) Dizziness

Dizziness is only a symptom and many diseases, especially cerebral diseases, can cause it.

Selected stimulating area: Dizziness and auditory area on both sides.

Treatment: Scalp acupuncture, applied once a day, can produce a satisfactory and quick cure of dizziness caused by functional diseases. It can also be used as a supplementary treatment for dizziness in patients with organic lesions.

Of the 200 cases of dizziness treated with scalp acupuncture, 116 were cured, accounting for 58 percent; 63 were greatly relieved, accounting for 31.5 percent; 19 were relieved to lesser degrees, accounting for 9.5 percent; and two did not show any effect. The total effective rate added up to 99 percent.

(3) Nervous Deafness

Nervous deafness is an auditory disorder due to injury of the cochlear nerve.

Selected stimulating area: Dizziness and auditory area on both sides.

Treatment: Scalp acupuncture, applied once a day, can restore hearing and cure deafness in some patients.

Of the 51 cases of plain nervous deafness treated with scalp acupuncture, 28 were cured, accounting for 54.9 percent; 13 were markedly relieved, accounting for 25.49 percent; four were relieved to a lesser degree, accounting for 7.8 percent; and six were did not show any effect.

Of the 33 cases of nervous deafness with tinnitus treated with scalp acupuncture, 11 were cured, accounting for 33.33 percent; 11 were apparently relieved, accounting for 33.33 percent; seven were relieved to a lesser degree, accounting for 21.21 percent; and four did not show any effect.

Case Report:

(1) Bilateral nervous deafness with tinnitus

Wang, male, 40 years old, from Yuncheng, Shanxi Province.

Chief complaint: Deafness of left ear for 12 years and deafness of right ear for six years.

Case history: One day in 1966, the patient suddenly developed tinnitus and impairment of hearing in his left ear, which made it difficult for him to talk with people face to face or on telephone. In 1973, he again lost hearing in the right ear after an attack of cold. Western and traditional Chinese medicine as well as routine acupuncture applied at the right Tinggong (SI 19) and Ermen (TE 21) acupoints all failed to produce any result. He came to seek treatment by scalp acupuncture on September 19, 1978.

Physical examination: The patient could not hear the ticktacks of watch in both ears or talk with people face to face. Both eardrums somewhat fell in.

Selected stimulating area: Dizziness and auditory area on both sides.

Treatment: Scalp acupuncture was applied once a day. After five rounds of treatment, the patient could hear the ticktacks of watch and hear phone calls with the left ear. After the ninth round of treatment, the patient could clearly hear TV sound three meters away from a TV set and clearly hear people talking.

(2) Right nervous deafness

Lan, female, 62 years old, from Dandong, Liaoning Province.

Chief complaint: Right deafness for 17 years.

Case history: One day in 1975, the patient suddenly felt there was something in her right ear, impairing the hearing and causing serious headache on the right side. She had tried many therapies all of which failed to produce any improvement to the symptoms. The condition became worse and worse until her right ear lost all hear one year after.

Physical examination: The patient had a clear state of mind and could express herself clearly. The hearing of the left ear was normal and that of the right ear was completely lost. She could not hear other people's shouting, if the left ear was blocked.

Diagnosis: Sudden and complete deafness of right ear.

Selected stimulating area: Dizziness and auditory area on both sides.

Treatment: Scalp acupuncture was applied once a day. After the first round of treatment, it seemed she could hear something. When the hearing of the right ear was measured on the next day before another round of treatment was given, she could hear the sound of hand clapping. After the second round of treatment, the hearing was much improved, and she could talk clearly with people standing on her right side while the left ear was blocked.

(4) Tinnitus

Tinnitus refers to the fact that people hear a continuous or intermittent sound which does not exist.

Selected stimulating area: Dizziness and auditory area on both sides.

Treatment: Scalp acupuncture, applied once a day, produces a more satisfactory therapeutic effect in patients with intermittent tinnitus than in those with continuous tinnitus. In some patients, the first round of treatment with scalp acupuncture can produce an apparent relief and several rounds can produce a complete cure.

Case Report:

Fan, female, 23 years old, from Wanrong County, Shanxi Province.

Chief complaint: Tinnitus in both ears for more than one month.

Case history: In early September 1992, the patient developed tinnitus because of insomnia. And the condition lasted for a month despite treatment with many drugs.

Physical examination: The patient had a clear state of mind. The hearing of both ears was normal. She said her tinnitus, which was continuous, was like the noise produced by a wheat mill.

Diagnosis: Bilateral tinnitus.

Selected stimulating area: Dizziness and auditory area on both sides.

Treatment: Scalp acupuncture was applied once a day. Some therapeutic effect was produced by the first round of treatment. After the third round of treatment, the tinnitus disappeared. Another six rounds of treatment were given to consolidate the therapeutic result.

(5) Injury of Vestibular Nerve

The function of vestibular nerve is to adjust the balance of the body (including the head, eyeballs, trunk and limbs) and the response of the body to speed acceleration. Under normal conditions, people rarely feel the activity of vestibular organs. They can only feel they are there when they are hindered or injured. The major manifestations of injury of the vestibular organs include vertigo, nystagmus, nausea and vomiting.

The vestibular nerves can be damaged by injection of streptomycin and gentamycin.

Selected stimulating area: Dizziness and auditory area on both sides.

Treatment: Scalp acupuncture, applied once a day, can remove the symptoms in some patients.

Case Report:

Lai, female, 51 years old, from Yuncheng, Shanxi Province.

Chief complaint: Vertigo due to injury of vestibular nerve by injection of streptomycin for five days.

Case history: The patient had for sometime suffered from chronic bronchitis and emphysema. Five days before, he went to a physician for cough, shortness of breath and chest pain. The physician prescribed to him intramuscular injections of penicillin and streptomycin, twice a day. Right after the third injection, she felt uncomfortable in the face and whole body. And after the injections for seven days, she felt serious dizziness, with an apparent unsteady gait to walk, just like a drunkard. The dizziness was even more serious when turning the head to the right side. She was accompanied to the hospital on June 4, 1978.

Physical examination: The patient could not walk by herself for the serious dizziness. She could not turn her head. Her horizontal nystagmus was positive. The hearing of the right ear was normal, and no tinnitus was felt.

Selected stimulating area: Dizziness and auditory area on both sides.

Treatment: Scalp acupuncture was applied once a day. The dizziness became less serious after the first round of treatment. After the second round of treatment, it was further relieved and the patient was able to walk independently. After the fourth round of treatment, the dizziness was completely gone, the nystagmus disappeared and she could come to the hospital by herself; yet, the turning of the head to the right still caused some dizziness. After the seventh round of treatment, all symptoms disappeared.

图书在版编目(CIP)数据

头针:英文/焦顺发著. —北京:外文出版社,1997
ISBN 7 – 119 – 01806 – X

Ⅰ.头… Ⅱ.焦… Ⅲ.头针疗法 – 英文 Ⅳ.R245.32

中国版本图书馆 CIP 数据核字 (95) 第 14639 号

头　针

焦顺发　著

责任编辑　刘文渊　刘春英

*

ⓒ外文出版社

外文出版社出版

（中国北京百万庄大街 24 号）

邮政编码 100037

北京外文印刷厂印刷

中国国际图书贸易总公司发行

（中国北京车公庄西路 35 号）

北京邮政信箱第 399 号　邮政编码 100044

1997 年(16 开)第 1 版

（英）

ISBN 7 – 119 – 01806 – X /R·129(外)

04800

14 – E – 3064S